HYPOTHESIS

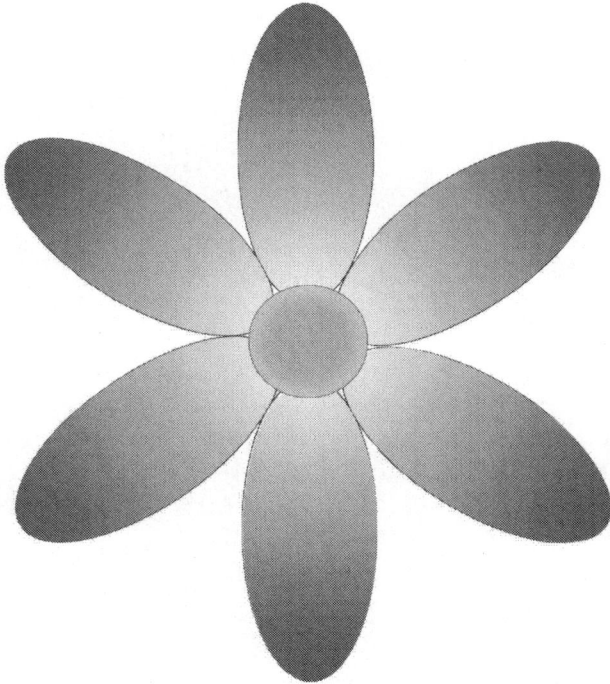

An HPV Healing Experiment

Teresa Marie Novak

Concept Bridges
2018

Table of Contents

Words from the Author

It's intriguing to me how closely related my greatest joys are to my most rooted fears. I have deep, heartfelt gratitude for the people who so generously offered their time and energy to help me transform many of my fears into previously unimaginable joy.

Karl Wiegers
Nicole Zdeb
Dr. Michael J. Lee, MD
Britt B. Steele
Dr. Karina Jarvela, ND
Dr. B. Gowey, NMD
The amazing women I had the privilege to interview
The early readers
My always supportive family and friends

Dedicated to

All those who through no effort of their own
just by being exactly who they are
are right now healing others

Sheri's story—many women's story

I was wiggling in my hairstylist's chair, feeling a bit unsettled, yet fully committed. I was confident Sheri had the skills to help me gracefully transition from bleached blond to my natural silver. I was expecting the usual chatty conversation, but Sheri was noticeably agitated.

Sheri: So, I am thinking about my two kiddos and I wanted to get long-term disability insurance, but was denied because I had a preexisting condition of HPV and cervical dysplasia.

Me: (eyes rolling about the insurance mess we are trying to live with) Really? Doesn't something like 80% of all people have HPV at some time? That's a preexisting condition now?

Sheri: Well, yes. I waited a year, because most of the time this just goes away on its own and if I re-Papped negative, I could get the insurance. But when I retested, the labs came back the same. I thought about it for a while, okay several months—because I didn't really want to face this. I had a hard time arriving at a decision and was hesitant because I understand even with LEEP [Loop Electrosurgical Excision Procedure] there was still a chance of the HPV and dysplasia returning. Medical treatments are a real trigger for my anxiety, and the doctor finally agreed I could have anesthesia during the procedure. So though it was hard for me emotionally and financially, I went ahead and followed my doctor's recommendation to get LEEP; and you know what *really* gets me? The labs came back, just today, completely negative!

Me: Oh, shit! You were fine by the time of the LEEP?

Sheri: See? You get me! After seeing the smoke rise from my body and choking on the smell of my own cervical flesh burning, all with the privilege of paying for the whole ordeal out of my own pocket, the last thing I wanted to hear was that there was nothing. He tried to spin it, like, aren't you glad we didn't find anything and you are free and clear of cancer? After going through everything I did, at this point I'd rather have the doctor report they found a nasty tumor and now it was completely removed. *At least then I would have something to be grateful for.*

Me: I also had HPV and cervical dysplasia. It's personal, so close to who we are as women. I am so sorry you had that experience.

But all the while, my inner voice was saying what I really wanted to say out loud, but couldn't—I knew it was too late to be helpful.

Sheri, your experience was one of my biggest fears, but a naturopath who's not more than two miles from this very shop specializes in treating HPV and cervical dysplasia. She helped me create my own path to healing—complete regression while keeping my cervix whole. There was more to my healing than naturopathy, though, a lot more. All of which I could have told you about sooner . . .

Part of my healing resulted in this wave of extreme self-acceptance I am experiencing right now—the very thing that brought me to you—to help me grow out my natural silver hair.

I found a way to detour the progressive threat of cervical cancer. My body knew exactly what to do. You see, my healing was mostly about winning the head-game and trusting myself.

Maybe it would have helped you too . . .

> **Each year in America**
> 20 million currently infected with HPV.
> Another 6 million people become newly infected.
> Cervical dysplasia affects between
> 250,000 and one million women.
> Half a million LEEP procedures.[1]
> LEEP overtreatment approximately
> 20% (~100,000 women).

What?

When it comes to HPV and cervical dysplasia, there's a lot of terminology and numbers. Studies are known to be inadequate and outdated, and there are many factors behind any given statistic.

Bottom line: there's a mountain of data points to wade through. It's a little mind-numbing. The information presented here is what I landed on based my own experience and choice-making.

I encourage you to do your own research and not take my word for it. The resources provided in the notes and index are a good starting place.

Pap

People often say "Pap" as short for Pap smear. This is a technique devised by George Nicholas Papanicolaou in the 1960s for a test carried out on a sample of cells from the cervix to check for abnormalities that may be indicative of cervical cancer. An HPV test can be done at the same time as a Pap, even with the same swab. When you get both tests, they call it 'co-testing'.[2]

HPV

The human papillomavirus (HPV) is the most common sexually transmitted disease, passed through genital contact. Approximately 20 million Americans are currently infected with HPV, and another 6 million people become newly infected each year. HPV has more than 100 types, of which at least 40 can infect the female genital tract. Most people who become infected with HPV do not know they have it, as the condition rarely causes symptoms or health problems. In many cases, the body's immune system clears HPV naturally within two years. The odds that a sexually active woman will be infected at least once in her lifetime with HPV are 80 percent.[3]

Cervical Dysplasia

Cervical dysplasia is caused by HPV and is the abnormal growth of cells on the surface of the cervix. These abnormal cells can be called lesions. This is considered to be a precancerous condition; hence it is often called stage-zero cervical cancer.[4] Cervical dysplasia lesions can regress (which means they shrink and may even disappear), persist (the lesions remain present but don't change), or progress to become a high-grade lesion or cervical cancer.[5] Cervical dysplasia affects between 250,000 and one million women throughout the United States every year.[6]

LEEP

LEEP stands for Loop Electrosurgical Excision Procedure. A small electrical wire loop is used to remove abnormal cells from the cervix[7] then the wound is burned to stop bleeding and prevent infection. Women with biopsy-confirmed cervical dysplasia routinely undergo LEEP, the go-to treatment for stage-zero cervical cancer. It's a procedure that is easily found on insurance plans and is a service provided by Planned Parenthood.[8]

> My gynecologist described LEEP as
> "common as sliced bread".

Given the propensity of HPV clearance over time, overtreatment of LEEP happens; like in the case of my hairdresser, Sheri.[9] Clinical studies tell us 20% of these procedures result in lab tests that indicate the cervix had no abnormal cells.

There is also an approach called "See-and-treat" that involves the diagnosis and LEEP treatment of cervical intraepithelial neoplasia (CIN) in a single visit. This is cited to reduces cost and clinic visits, loss to follow-up, and patient anxiety. Overtreatment rates range from 4 to 18%.[10]

Though many publications mention "there are no data to suggest that overtreatment is harmful",[11] after hearing many women describe their experience in considering and undergoing a LEEP procedure, it seems their definition of harmful could use some refinement.

What do you believe?

What if based on your last Pap or STI screening, your doctor tells you to schedule a time to have a surgical procedure that removes part of your body because you might develop cancer? And that part of your body is your cervix?

Do you believe:

- Given the chance, your body heals itself?

- The standard "Watch and wait" treatment guideline lacks currency and is insensitive to your needs?

- Your thoughts affect your health, but you are not quite sure how to manage that?

- You want to take charge of your own wellness, and you like to assess information and decide for yourself, but you need a little guidance in how to make decisions?

- Increased awareness could help reduce the social shame associated with HPV and cervical dysplasia and increase loving support for women facing this diagnosis?

If your head is nodding *yes* to any of these, the information in this book may be exactly what you are seeking.

Could you use tips and resources for how to win the head-game associated with the HPV/cervical dysplasia diagnosis? Things like:

- Meditation that includes visualization and gratitude

- Making space for joy in your life

- Tips for making it through naturopathic cervical topical treatments and still feel 'normal'? Including how to keep your sex life going strong?

Curious? Getting that 'yes' feeling?

What if I told you that you can heal yourself?

You can design your own treatment plan, and for that matter, right now, through absolutely no effort of your own, you are healing others.

In this book, I'll teach you, through engaged observation, how to accept things as they are and use that as an advantage in designing solutions you can bring alive, right now, to transform yourself and others. I will step you through these things, first by sharing my experience as an example. Along the way you will hear the voices and perspectives of others who have been through the same choice-making. Then you'll learn a process for defining your own healing hypothesis, conduct your own healing experiment and reveal conclusions about yourself and your world that I predict are beyond your wildest expectations.

PART 1

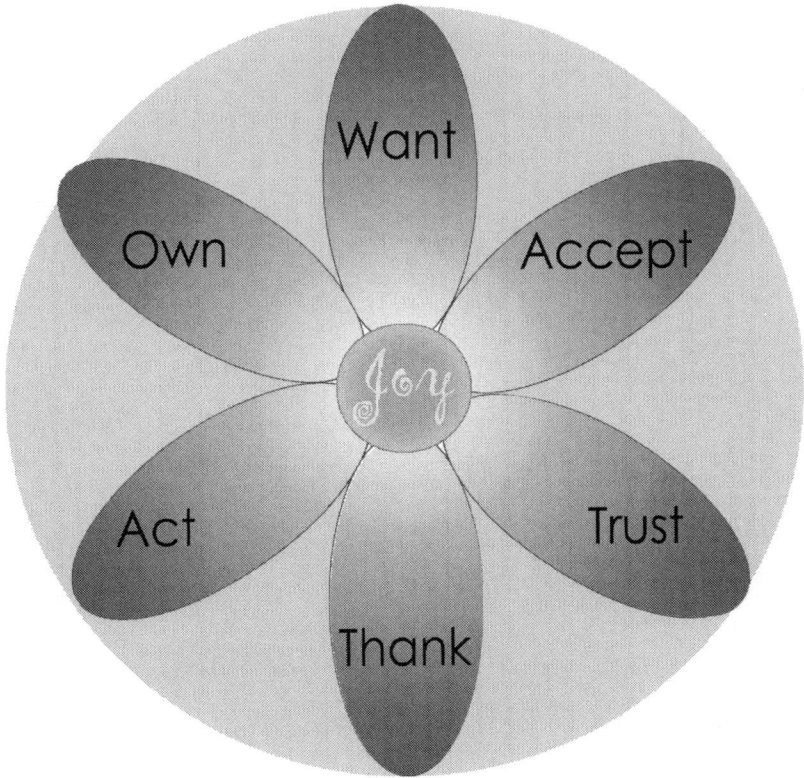

How I healed myself (spoiler/no spoiler)

My formal education was in physics and mathematics. As it turned out, I made a career of helping people define their problems and desires. Scientific method, decision models, process flows; that's where I feel at home. I used these methods thousands of times in system analysis; that's how I became an expert in creating and implementing processes that bring about change.

In my own HPV/cervical dysplasia journey, I applied what I learned during more than twenty years in software engineering to define my own personal experiment in self-healing. The process I used is at its core the scientific method.[12] I augmented it with explicit mention of the power of heart and mind, but the process is essentially the same.

One Process—Infinite Possibilities

Because everyone is unique and everyone's situation is different, there won't be a single solution that works for everyone. There are infinite ways to heal and you will have a chance to design the one way that is perfect for you. That said, there *is* one process that can guide everyone in choice-making. I modeled this process as an infinity flower.

Each petal is a step in the process; joy is always at the center, like a propeller, moving healing forward.

This can be a guide for *any* problem-solving really: but for our purposes now, this process will be used to define your own personal experiment in self-healing. I reference the infinity flower throughout the book, to emphasize where we are in the process.

> It's really a series of decisions, which establish a commitment.

These decisions don't have to happen in any given order, and you don't have to have all the decisions made before you begin to take action.

As a guide, however, start at the top with what you know and then go around the clock.

For anyone facing hard choices I offer this: it doesn't matter how old you are, how much the odds are against you, or how tough the social pressure and mental angst may seem.

> If you create your own path based on joy and gratitude, then do what it takes to keep moving forward, you will realize your vision.

I will guide you through this process first as I experienced it in my own story and then again as *you* define *your own* healing hypothesis, so you can conduct your own healing experiment. If your experience is anything like mine, you will reveal discoveries about your own power to heal that are beyond your wildest expectations.

My story

My path was all about keeping my cervix whole, which started in the wake of an unsettling diagnosis of high-risk HPV plus cervical dysplasia. My Western male gynecologist said in his thirty-year practice he'd *never* seen women my age avoid cancer progression without surgical intervention. My female naturopath said in her twenty years of practice, *100%* of her clients regressed.

Who to trust? The doctor covered by my insurance with federally and scientifically approved methods who has *zero* track record of healing a person like me, or the doctor who includes what many consider pseudo-science in her practice and yet successfully healed hundreds of women like me.

That's when I made the decision to trust myself!

This is how I healed myself from stage zero cervical cancer, and the steps I took to reach full regression—at age fifty.

Summary of my healing experiment

The treatment plan I designed for myself required a commitment to incorporate alternative medicine into my everyday life. I approached this as my own personal experiment in self-healing, and measured my progress with standard cervical cancer screenings.

1. Naturopathic treatments

- eating to control and reduce inflammation
- probiotics and other supplements found to build the immune system, fight viruses and clear skin
- natural topical treatments (to the cervix) found to stimulate a healing response
- treating root cause of other persistent and recurrent infections around my body

2. Yoga practices

- breathing and moving (primarily pawanmuktasana[13])
- meditation (creating a vision of gratitude and letting go of what no longer serves me)
- mantra (Om Gam Ganapataye Namaha)

3. Screenings

Cancer progression screenings according to the American Congress of Obstetricians and Gynecologists (ACOG) schedule of Well-Woman ages 40–64 and Cervical Cancer Screening ages 30–65.

- 1 year Pap with HPV follow-up for positive lab findings

- Colposcopy with punch biopsy for positive lab findings

- 3-month Pap/HPV follow-up for positive visual and/or lab findings (repeat cycle)

- 6-month Pap/HPV follow-up for first negative lab findings

- 12-month Pap/HPV follow-up for second negative lab findings

This plan isn't for everybody, but it was perfect for me

I will be the first to say, the treatment plan outlined isn't for everybody. In truth, it may be only for me—to date, I have not heard of anyone in my similar condition replicating this plan and getting the same results. What were the results, you may ask? So not only am I clear of HPV and cervical dysplasia, I no longer use topical steroids in my ears (did that for twenty years!), the recurrent urinary tract infections I struggled with for years are gone, bacterial vaginosis is now a rare occurrence, hemorrhoids that started after I gave birth in my twenties are under control and, like I mentioned to my naturopath with a smile, when the toe wart is gone we will know I am healed (and it's gone). Too much information? There are, of course, even more incredible results, but you will see that unfold in the rest of the story!

That said, I am curious—as you read this book and design your own healing experiment, if it ends up sounding a lot like mine, please contact me! Even if your plan is something *completely different*, I would *still* love to hear about your own healing experiment.*

---

* Seriously, I would love to hear from you. See my Facebook page Terrie Novak – Author, my Instagram theterrienovak, or just email me: terrie.concept@gmail.com.

To that point, the main purpose of this book is to walk you through a process of designing your own, personalized treatment plan and while we are at it, throw in a lot of encouragement and love along the way!

It's my hope that by sharing my real-life example, people facing HPV and cervical dysplasia will feel empowered to face their situation and avoid some stress or confusion associated with scheduling procedures they are uncomfortable with.

Disclaimer

I am in no way qualified to give medical, naturopathic or yoga advice. I encourage you to do your own research and engage with professionals associated with actions you choose to go forward with.

I will share with you the findings of my own research, and maybe save you some time or anxiety by sharing resource references and tips. One of my greatest resources was the words of experience from women just like me (like us!). Women who have faced these same choices. Just people you meet in your everyday life; like your sister, lover, colleague, teacher or hairdresser. I am so grateful that many have agreed to share their voices and perspectives in this book.

It's about awareness of options and the empowerment of making decisions. I will be with you every step of the way by providing a guide for working through what can be a tough choice-making process.

My investigations and discoveries are given to you as a guide. Each chapter offers my personal story as an example and then tangible steps and resources to help *you decide* the best path for you.

At the time when I was going through this, my approach was to be my own human experiment.

Like all things, it starts with a decision.

For me, I decided my cervix was worth fighting for.

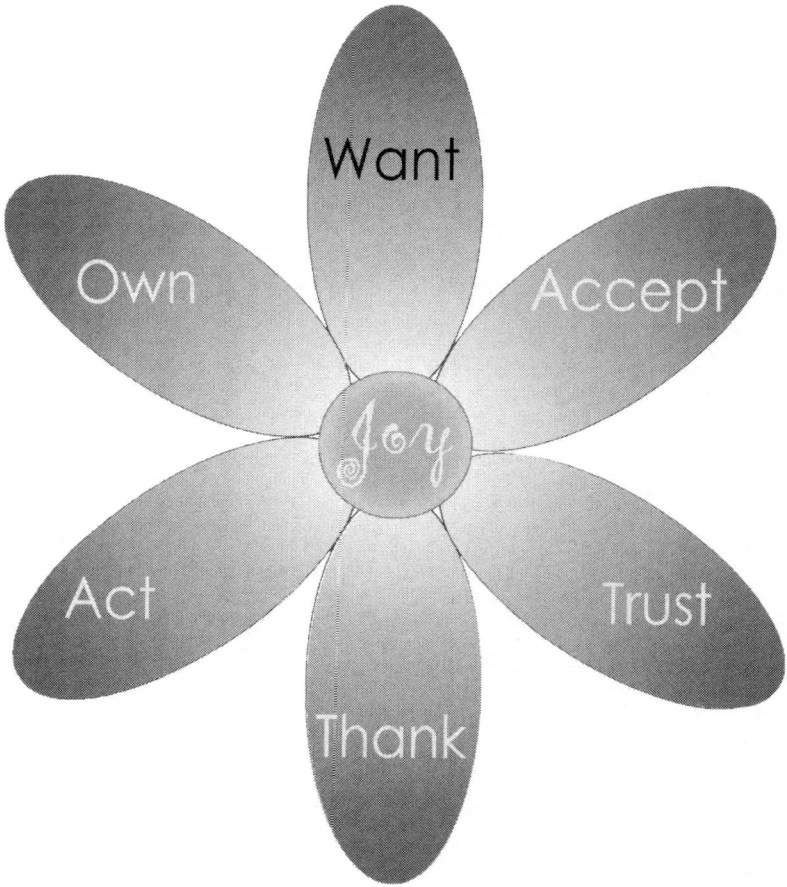

Diagnosis

Everyone seems to remember the diagnosis moment; I have heard many stories akin to remembering what you were doing that day of the 9/11 attacks. With something as personal as your cervix being threatened, we usually think of what's going on with our relationships.

> *For some reason, I am remembering this time period, it was after my Mother passed away so there was an added sense of aloneness and fear.*
> *—College student's first STI experience,*
> *a cryosurgery patient*

At first startling and confusing, then hot and expansive, like a slap: I got the cervical dysplasia slap in that same appointment room where over the course of a year I had two Paps and one colposcopy, so definitely not my favorite room. They do a good job of being as friendly and warm as possible, but the items in the room are still clinical (the IUD models are informative, but creepy) and damn, why can't they ever make the temperature warm-ish? The stirrups, uggh. I am always slightly entertained when the nurse says, "Sit wherever you want."

Me: So, it doesn't seem to be going away. What do I do now?

Gyn: (without a second of hesitation) You can go ahead and schedule a LEEP procedure with reception on your way out.

Me: Is this an out-patient thing?

Gyn: Oh, yes, just right here in the office. *It's as common as sliced bread.*

Me: What is LEEP exactly?

Gyn: (shaping his hands to mimic a cervix, indicating how much length was involved) It's an electric current that takes off about a half-inch of the cervix, removing the abnormal cells.

Me: (now feeling my gut tightening thinking about cutting off a half-inch of my body, down there, in there) So, I understand what I have is not cancer, right? So why would I do this now?

Gyn: In my thirty years of practice, *I've never seen a woman your age regress.*

> *I have a body that's aging. I have a body that's growing older. And the older my body gets the more I'm going to come up against this stuff, so, I need to do this right.*
>
> —*LEEP patient*

Wait, what?

I am *too old* to heal from this? Ever?

I stood up and mumbled something resembling the tones of thank you and goodbye and bolted past the receptionist with some strange degree of guilt and shame for ignoring the opportunity to expediently schedule the common-as-sliced-bread procedure. I slinked into the safe and snug sanctum of my car and hunkered down with my friend Google.

Me: What is cervical dysplasia and HPV?

Google: Abnormal cells on cervix, stage zero cancer

Me: Treatments.

Google: cone biopsy, LEEP, Cold-knife

Me: (WTF? Cold-knife?) What is LEEP?

Google: pain medications, low-voltage electrical current, wire removing abnormal areas of cervix, 5-30 percent fail rate.[14] Want to see pictures? Video?

Me: Did I just get prescribed a treatment that can fail one-third of the time?

First, I felt like there was nothing wrong with me. Essentially, physically, I felt fine. Better than fine, actually. Second, tell me again why I would remove a portion of my cervix when I felt fine? Jesus, was this my life now? Starting the downhill progression of screenings and treatments?

Head still spinning and feeling a bit like I was doing something wrong by not following my doc's advice to schedule a date for LEEP, I gave myself permission to take some time to clear my head. A confusion and investigation period: two months—to look things up, talk with some people and *then* make a choice about treatment. Everything from there would be done in an orderly fashion, right?

> *Keep having screenings until they show up with cancer just isn't a good answer. Even she (primary care doctor) doesn't think it's a good answer, but that's all she's got.*
> *—on "Watch and Wait" from a 27-year-old monitoring HPV for 10 years with annual Paps*

Freak-out

Reaction is unique to each person. However, in my conversations with women facing treatment choices associated with cervical dysplasia, some degree of freaking out seems to be something we all have in common.

> *If this piece of me is causing such problems, why don't I just have a hysterectomy and get it over with?*
>
> *—LEEP patient, when describing her freak-out moment*

I kept tripping over my gyn's cavalier bedside manner: as common as sliced bread, for God's sake. There is certainly a culture of insufficient concern for this women's issue. Men can't get cancer from this, after all, right?

This is about my *cervix*, it's *personal*. I don't see anything simple or everyday about it. I don't want to pursue any treatment that makes me feel medically underserved as a person.

My internal voice of reaction didn't stop there . . .

Shamed me: Should I not talk about this to anyone?

Analyzing me: Is that shame I am feeling? This is, after all, in part caused by a sexually transmitted disease. Will people think I am not a good person?

Hover-Mom me: How will this affect my kids? My parents? I want to be a role model for my kids and my family. I want them to know this challenge I am facing is not a secret, nor something to sweep under the rug, nor something to be ashamed of. *I want my family to be at peace when they think about my health and well-being.*

Bad-idea me: Should I hide it from them?

Unworthy me: Do I deserve this? I *have* chosen to have multiple partners as a lifestyle, after all . . .

Judging me: Was that wrong? Maybe remaining single and continuing to pursue intimate relationships really is too risky.

Analyzing me: Why am I avoiding the doctor's treatment suggestion? Am I foolish to not just follow the most conservative/aggressive treatment plans to avoid progression of cancer? I am, after all, 'old'. I am certainly not going to have a baby anymore. Am I holding on too tight to body parts that just don't really matter anymore?

Jumping-to-conclusions me: Will I never have pleasurable sex again?[15] It took me fifty years to discover cervical orgasms and I am not giving that up without a fight. The intimacy in my current relationship is a huge part of what makes me feel alive. I know there are countless new kinds of intimacies yet to surface and explore and yet, I want to savor sexual activities I've found that make me feel truly alive as long as I can, and for now, that involves keeping my cervix.

Crystal-ball me: Should I start mentally, physically and financially preparing for the progression of having my body parts removed? The likelihood of chemo?

Conspiracy-theory me: Why do they even call it 'stage zero cancer'? That term seems like an evil plot to brainwash a large number of women into predetermining for themselves that things may go in a bad direction so they seek out extra screenings and services that feed into the corrupt insurance system. Is that why he didn't offer even a single alternative treatment option?

Freak-out me: Is it possible to stop worrying about this? Ever? Is this just who I am now? A person going down the path of dealing with cancer?

I spent the next few days freaking out, pressing into my fearful thoughts. Nothing very productive came of that initial reaction inside my head. The breakthrough to the other side of freaking out happened when I began to reach out to others, and state my hopes and fears out loud.

Say it out loud

After a day of Google searches that followed my random thoughts and reactions, it was time for date night with my primary partner. We were part of a polyamorous triad for just less than a year and we dedicated one day a week for each other. A day to focus just on our being together, no matter what shape that came in. With this simple commitment to each other we had already grown to know and love each other deeply. That day, I texted him to cancel our date, something I knew was against our time-commitment agreement.

Butterfly: (text message Me) I had something upsetting come up and I need to be alone for a while and think about it. I think it's best, just this one time, we cancel our day.

Bear: What's important is that I am with you, I want to be with you no matter how you are. There is no such thing as canceling our day together. <heart emoticons>

Butterfly: (after an exhale of annoyance) Okay, then, but it's a stay-in night.

Here's the thing: I hadn't told him about my previous high-risk HPV lab results (those that did *not* show cervical dysplasia). Why?

When I explicitly asked my gyn if I should disclose the high-risk HPV lab result with intimate partners he said, "It's not really anything you need to talk about." So, I didn't.

Living a sex-positive lifestyle, open communication and frequent screenings were expectations of everyone we participated with in consensual intimate activities. But high-risk HPV, which typically is something that resolves on its own, didn't seem important to mention—until now.

I was relieved and annoyed he still wanted our date night. I needed his support and comfort which I wasn't sure he would be able to deliver once I retroactively disclosed my HPV situation—now all wrapped up with my latest diagnosis and new fears. I knew I'd be testing the waters of our relationship, to see if he would stick around for the potentially never-ending journey of dealing with this.

Bear: what do you need to talk about?

Me: (chin quivering, no words forming)

Bear: (just holding me) Let's get a shower.

And just like a loving parent comforting a wailing baby, he turned on the sound, rhythmic feel, and warmth of the shower, stepping in with me, holding me. Waiting for words to come.

Me: (blubbering out some word groups) Gynecologist . . . HPV . . . cervix . . . dysplasia . . . old immune system . . . LEEP . . . hysterectomy . . . chemo . . .

Me: I don't know how this is going to go. I don't know what sex could be like during or after this, and that's just the sex part. I have no idea about all the rest.

Bear: (while kissing my forehead): *We will find a way.*

And just by being who he is, he started my healing.

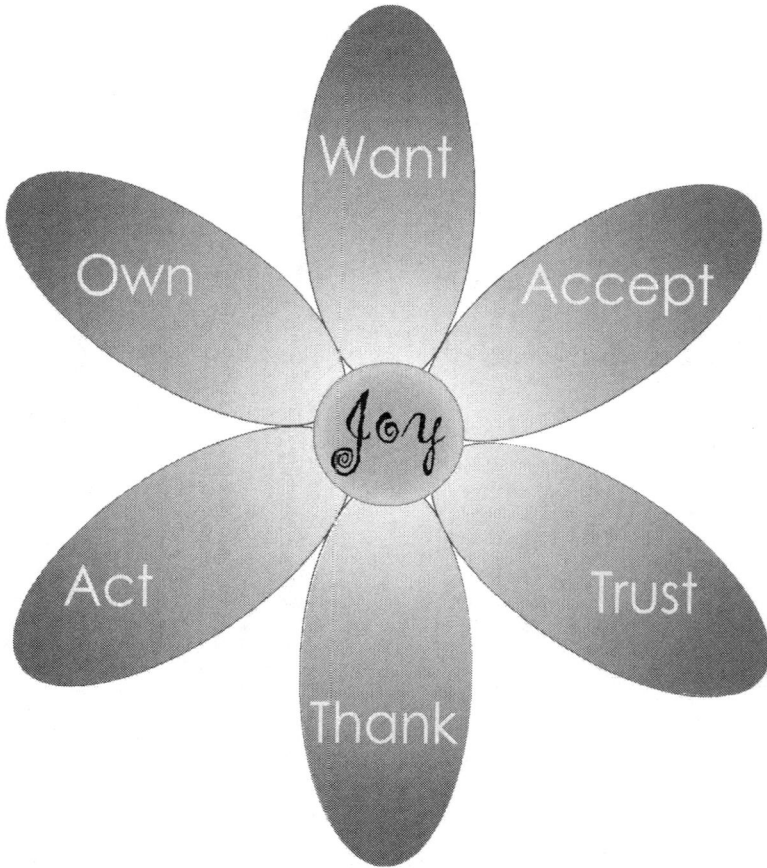

Fear of the last chance

Like the many women I had the opportunity to meet and chat with who have experienced this same challenge, I too was overwhelmed with the feeling of 'this is my last chance'.

> *Is this the universe telling me I shouldn't have a baby?*
> *—38-year-old LEEP patient*

Finding my joy in fear

In just the last several years I discovered joy in doing new exciting things with my mind and body. The explorations involved being awake, open and in the moment, and it was all delicious. I couldn't remember a time I felt more alive—except maybe when I was a teenager. My heart felt it was finally allowed to shine. Generous, loving people and new experiences were consistently arriving at my doorstep, and I felt ready to greet them.

I explored yoga and dancing. I entered a polyamorous triad. I began communicating my feelings and discoveries with those I loved: my kids, my family, my friends. Even if it wasn't always comfortable, I strived for loving honesty. I committed to creating the time and space for all this to occur.

Then, with the HPV/cervical dysplasia diagnosis, came the looming thoughts of a progression of treatments that may lie ahead of me. I feared all this would push aside these newly discovered joys from ever being accessible to me again.

I felt compelled to get in *one last thing*, before it was too late; something I had been looking forward to for a very long time . . .

For me, this one last thing turned out to be one special yoga pose: the pose that brought me into yoga years ago, a constant inspiration: the eight-angle pose.[16]

If only I could master this pose, I would have *something*. Something before the big decline began.

I knew I could count on my yoga teacher—she mentioned in her online forums that we could reach out to her at any time. Over the years I've followed her teachings, I found that everything she said, no matter how hippy or too good to be true it sounded, was in the end something tangible I could count on. So, completely out of character for me, I *called her*. Yep, dialed her home phone. I figured I could go to her Wednesday class downtown and catch her for a few minutes of personal advice in between classes.

Yoga studio

The downtown yoga studio is trendy and always buzzing with beautiful people with mats in tote, grabbing shoes, standing in line for the vegan food and the juice bar. It's surprisingly noisy for a yoga studio and has the earthy smell of cooked beans, steamed kale and sweat.

Me: (feeling suddenly self-conscious about the several frantic voice messages I left her, and my stalking her in between classes) I have this cervical dysplasia, stage zero cancer, and I don't know what to do about it. I just want to have something, something before I can't have it anymore, and I was wondering do you think it's possible for me to learn how to do the eight-angle pose in ten or twelve weeks?

Yoga teacher: (so beautiful as to ignore my crazy, blurting, nonsensical train of thought) You need to breathe.

Me: Yes, yes, I know I should breathe, but do you think you could teach me? Do you think I could do that?

Yoga teacher: What I mean is, cancer can't live with oxygen.

You need to breathe.

Okay. So, I am a scientist at heart and by training: physics, math, engineering, yada-yada. Research-based findings, scientific method, Bill Nye, Ms. Frizzle, I love that stuff. I played 'pediatrician' instead of 'house' when I was a kid. My first tattoo is the equation that represents the Mandelbrot set.

> The notion of alternative medicine just wasn't something I ever seriously considered.

And though I have grown to trust my teacher and her expertise in this area, this honestly sounded pretty over-the-top hippy for me. We arranged for me to come to the next week's class where she would include in her lesson preparatory movements for Astavakrasana and she would introduce me to some pranayama, which is Sanskrit for "breath control", where prana means "life force".

There was a cold wind to fight as I went to my car after that. I was twirling in my mind why she wouldn't just say "yes, you can" or "no, that's impossible". I wanted something a little more black and white and a little less tie-dye.

And yet, as I reflected on her suggestion that yogic breathing practices could help me, *I felt this huge sigh of relief (yep, a deep-to-the soul-exhale, it was like that)*. A warm wave of hope came over me, which was a welcome contrast to the feelings I had when it was suggested I fry off part of my cervix.

She had introduced pranayama in her classes I had attended some years ago. I found these techniques difficult and they often left me dizzy and uncomfortable. I had respect for the ancient practice, but no understanding of it.

Her notion of breathing to heal immediately felt like something I wanted. It resonated with me. I knew this was something I could hold onto.

The idea that there were options in treating these pre-cancerous cells turned my fear into curiosity.

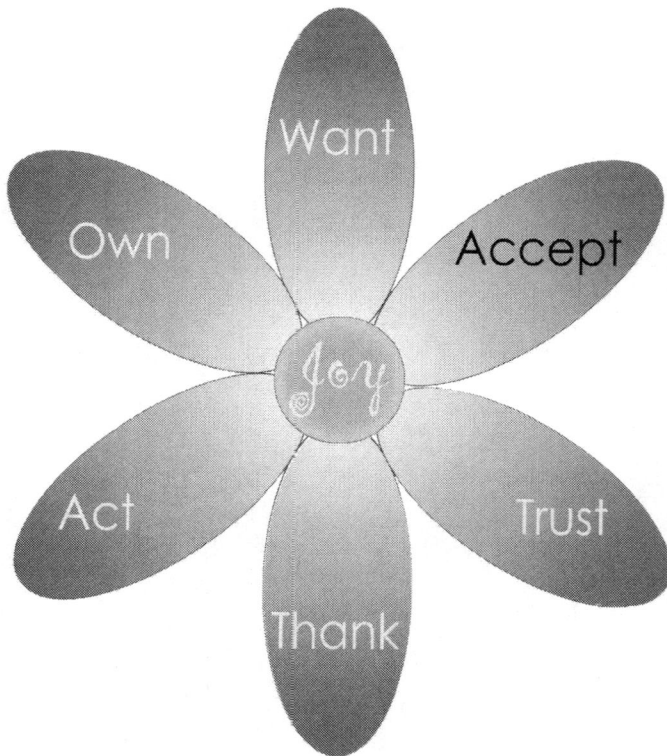

Now that I'm curious . . . Fear, come with me

Thinking about how I could up my yoga game, I figured if I was willing to take something like breathing as a 'real' way to heal the cervical dysplasia, what else is out there that I could consider a viable alternative treatment to LEEP?

I had a colleague who swore by her positive results with homeopathic treatments. Her descriptions of the 'remedies' honestly did sound like snake-oil to me. I decided to have another conversation with my friend Google about alternative medicine.

Me: cervical dysplasia alternative treatment options

Google: 355,000 results—reversing cervical dysplasia naturally, dysplasia healed without surgery

Me: Wait, what? *This isn't obscure.* Why didn't I see or hear of any of this before? Cervical dysplasia natural treatments in my local area.

Google: State licensed naturopath[17] specializing in gynecology, HPV protocols, and cervical dysplasia, only 13 miles away. Want a map?

Me: (dialing the phone number for an appointment) What? Only twenty minutes from my house?

Naturopath's Office

The naturopath's office was in a part of town with triangle streets and that got me off to a frustrating start on this adventure. It didn't help that the house-converted-to-office was nestled between a massage studio with Tarot card displays in the front window and a skin care shop that offered facials and had threatening parking signage.

Despite all that, I entered and was greeted by a smiling receptionist who looked genuinely happy to be working there and serving people, which was pretty different from my primary care facility, where the receptionist basically herded people through, and processed co-pays in take-a-number fashion. There were plants throughout the office and I was offered to help myself to hot herbal tea. Glancing at the tea bags, I Googled 'tumeric' and decided to pass for now. It felt calm there. I wasn't expecting it, but I started to enjoy a moment of peace. After having my height, weight, temperature and blood pressure measured, the doctor soon invited me into her office—which was painted bright yellow.

Me: You have treated cervical dysplasia and HPV before? Even for women my age?

Naturopathic doc: Yes, many times, hundreds.

Me: What is the typical outcome?

Naturopathic doc: In my twenty years of practice, all my patients regressed.

Me: (assessing if she was just being rather loose with words) You mean 100% of the patients you have treated for cervical dysplasia have totally cleared?

Naturopathic doc (now *my* naturopathic doc): Yes.

She continued to interview me. Asking about everything. I wanted to be as honest and complete in my answers as possible so she had a full understanding of what she was dealing with. I wanted her to be in a good position to make a well-informed treatment plan.

My description of myself included: multiple partners both male and female, taking oral contraceptives for well over fifteen years, drinking one alcoholic beverage most days, over-working and under-sleeping, inconsistent exercise, irregular bowel movements about every two days for pretty much my entire adult life, chronic infections including bacterial vaginosis and UTIs, eating generally on the go what was convenient and easy to grab.

> By the time I said all that, I felt like I had the words "viruses welcome here" stamped on my forehead.

She prompted me for details of any kind of symptom or feeling I had in my body or mind no matter the severity or longevity of the issue. She had recommendations for every topic, which she offered to me so I could *choose* what I wanted to commit to doing. I actually felt like she really cared about me and was personally invested in my healing. Like we were partners in this. She helped me to articulate where I was now *and* to say out loud how I wanted this all to end.

> What I heard come out of my mouth was not only the beginning of my vision of wellness, but the beginning of me accepting me.

After almost a full hour of conversation, I stood up from her desk with a treatment plan in hand (literally a two-page typed document) we both agreed would be doable and would get me the results I was seeking.

I checked out with the receptionist to find my visit was completely covered by my insurance (why didn't I know about that?), except the supplements were not, however I was able to put them on my employer provided Flex Spending account. For the topical treatments, I had to go to a compounding pharmacy (what is that?).

I drove home on autopilot. A bit stunned really that this whole world was available to me and I had no idea.

Investigation Summary

The two-month investigation time agreement I made with myself was over. It was time for choice-making and commitment.

I summed up what I had learned so far:

- I have cervical dysplasia and HPV that my body isn't clearing on its own. That has a probability of leading to cancer, so I have decided to treat it (somehow).

- The gyn resolved *zero cases* like mine without surgery and recommended LEEP to remove abnormal cells. His treatment recommendations are guided by the standard ACOG screening, which he follows on the conservative side.

- The naturopath, licensed to prescribe everything the Western doctor can *plus* homeopathic and naturopathic treatments, knows she's *healed 100% of women* like me. Her recommended treatments involve use of supplements and natural topical herb cocktails applied to my cervix that are not covered by my insurance.

- My yoga teacher, who already has my trust, recommends the healing power of ancient breathing and moving practices.

- My partner knows we will find a way and recommends we keep loving each other.

I could hardly recognize all this as something in *my* life, yet here it was.

I reached out for advice and advice was given.

Now it was up to me to decide. I decided to take my health and healing into my own hands—I would take *the advice I sought out*. It was time to be *all in*.

Hypothesis—an educated guess

My hypothesis: if I trust my intuition, their expertise and allow in the joy of the support of those I love, I will be healthy.

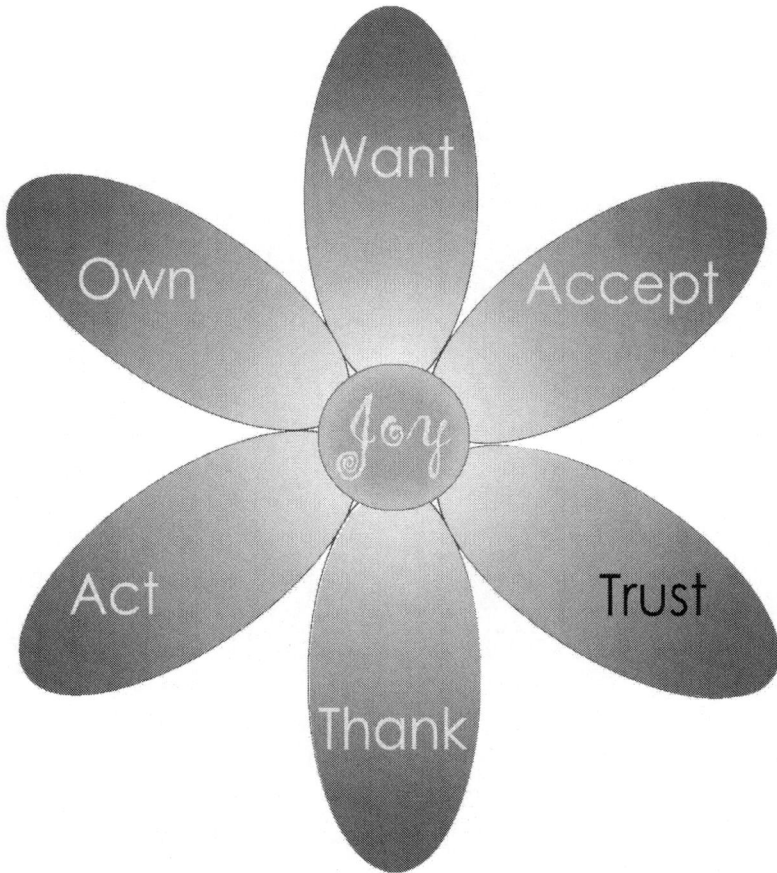

My healing experiment

I promised myself to be my own experiment: to take ownership of my healing and my health. I committed to testing my hypothesis by conducting procedures exactly as described by the experts I engaged and by validating the results with scientifically approved measurements.

This became my plan of action, my path to healing.

Procedure #1: Naturopathic medicine.
Follow the practices prescribed by the naturopath. Trust her to guide me through treatments that enable my body to heal itself by simultaneously stimulating and supporting my immune system.

Procedure #2: Yoga practice.
Follow the practices taught by my yoga teacher. Trust her to help me train my mind and nervous system to accept all healing energy and let go of all that is no longer serving me.

Procedure #3: Thank-you.
This procedure was not defined during my early investigation period, but it did surface during the inner reflection that was an important part of the yoga practice. I chose to include it in my experiment so I could test the contribution of gratitude, not knowing at the time that this would lead to an amazingly profound conclusion.

Measure: Cervical cancer screening.
It was important to me to have a non-biased measurement in my experiment. I trusted my gyn to let me know if I needed to escalate to a

more conventional treatment. If the screening indicated a possibility for regression, I would decline surgery. If I didn't regress, the mainstream treatment protocols remained available as a solid backup. If I did regress, my hypothesis would be correct!

Joy: I promise to keep doing those things that bring me joy. This requires reserving space to be with my kids, family and friends, continuing to share open communication and trust in their loving response.

I trust my partner to love me and encourage me to keep joy in my life, no matter how this turns out.

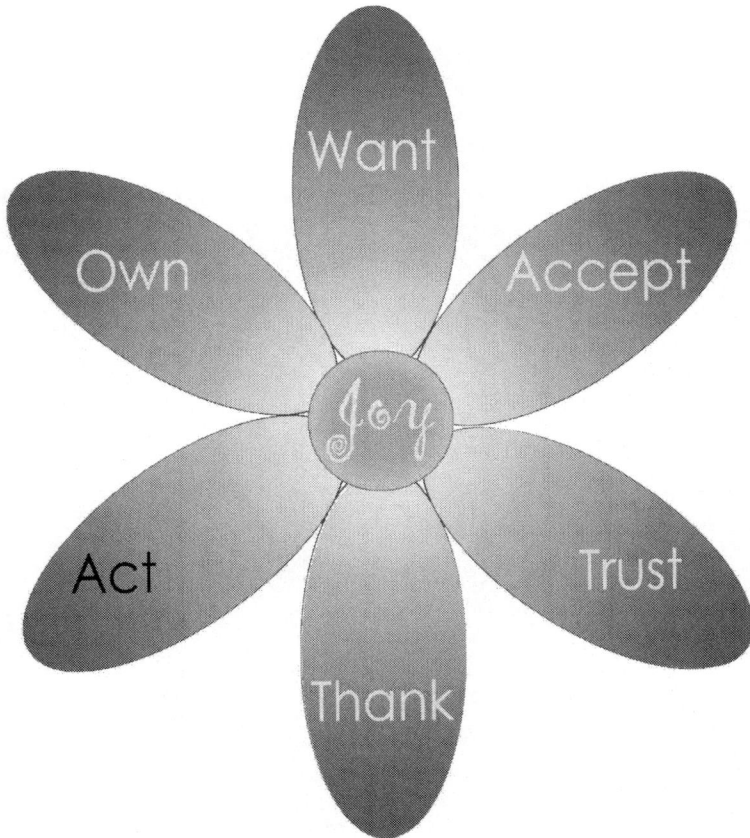

Procedure 1: Naturopathic medicine

There are two components to achieving regression. The first is to clear the HPV virus, which in large part is treated with boosting the immune system. The second part is to clear the cervix of abnormal cells, which is basically accomplished by destroying them.

Just like any prescription, I needed to find the treatments that I responded to best. For me, there was a lot of trial and error in both areas. My naturopath attributes that to my stubborn nature, which kind of made me laugh, but at the same time, I had to agree.

Anti-inflammatory eating

To give my immune system a chance to focus on getting rid of the HPV, it needed to stop having to spend so much energy on reacting to food sensitivities. As far as I knew at the time, I wasn't really allergic to any foods.

I knew that eating bread left me with a 'stone in my gut' feeling, so I stopped eating bread years ago to avoid the discomfort. I also knew that milk gave me terrible gas, so I quit drinking milk. I experimented with many diets with weight control as the primary driver and they all 'worked' for me more or less: everything from Atkins Diet to green-juice fasting. I gave up fast-food already (thank you Super-Size Me). I was vegan for a couple of years (after watching documentaries on the current practices in meat production) which, according to my Western doctor, may have been contributing to the recurrent UTIs and skin infections that had cropped up; he suggested following the Paleo diet and taking up Cross-Fit. So I put meat and eggs back in my diet and though I did lose weight, the chronic infections remained, as did the fact I only pooped a few times a week.

My body seemed flexible about dietary changes, so when the naturopath suggested taking an allergy test (blood from finger pricks) and removing some foods from my diet, I was ready to give it a go.

Even though I was ready to deal with false positives which the blood test is notorious for, I was a little surprised at the rather long and all-encompassing list of foods that came back on the test.

Nearly half the report was dedicated to all the kinds of eggs I showed allergic reaction to: chicken egg yolks, chicken egg whites, goose egg yolks, goose egg whites, etc.... you think of an egg description, it was on the results list.

Bananas was at the very top of the list. This seemed weird at first, but once I thought about it, I realized I don't really like bananas and only ate them when I felt I needed to boost vitamins, and during those times I always felt lousy. So this actually made really great sense to me. I was genuinely happy to think I wouldn't buy or eat another banana!

Some things were not as straightforward—whey protein and baker's and brewer's yeast.

I started making a list of foods I would avoid based on the 'starter' information that the blood test provided.

- No eggs, whey protein or soy
- No bananas, pineapple, cranberries or almonds
- No wheat or spelt, baker's yeast or brewer's yeast

Also, no dairy, baked goods, protein/energy bars, meat substitutes, shellfish or bubbly drinks.

In addition to that the naturopath added:

- No alcohol
- No caffeine

Good-bye convenience and pleasure eating.

Hello conscious eating for my body's nutrition.

In reflection, this all made perfect sense. I didn't need the naturopath or the allergy test to tell me these things, I simply needed to listen to and accept what my body has been telling me for years (decades, right?). Remember throwing up on bananas when you were pregnant? Remember going the emergency room based on a gut-wrenching panic attack founded on eating a bad egg salad sandwich? Remember having to quit the coffee club at work because your stomach was wrecked every day by 3pm? Remember ruining every trip to Mexico with diarrhea that started just after the first traditional piña colada by the pool vacation kick-off party drink? Remember the immediacy of zits showing up on your chin after eating Mom's baking?

What was preventing me from listening to my body?

Accepting my body. I needed to trust and respect the way it reacts to take care of me and let that be right, good and okay.

For that matter, neither a blood test nor historic episodes are needed to try out an elimination diet. One way to go about it is to take two to three weeks off from eating the most common allergy-inducing foods: milk, eggs, fish, shellfish, tree nuts, peanuts, wheat and soybeans. That is darn close to what I ended up doing anyway.

Procedure for anti-inflammatory eating

The only way I would be able to conduct this eating experiment was to:

1. Make space in my life for the time to shop for, prepare, and cook meals, and to store ingredients.

2. Shop for whole organic foods. Focus on fresh produce.

3. Read ingredient labels. If I bought anything with a label, I read it. If it contained any trace amount or any warning

about the foods I was avoiding, I just put it straight back on the shelf.

4. Don't rush prep-time. I clean and chop a lot of veggies! Taking my time is for safety reasons as well as for an opportunity to focus on imbuing my healing intent right into my food and for feeling gratitude for how it will nourish and heal me.

5. Cook and store food to retain its highest nutritional value. That includes using non-toxic cookware and storage containers.

6. Replace restaurants with grocery stores where I could eat whole prepared dishes that are mostly veggies and lean meats.

Materials list

- Veggie brush. I replaced a lot of peeling with buying organic and scrubbing, so I could maximize the opportunity to absorb nutrients.

- Santuko knife. Chopping with a knife with a straight edge is so much easier for me!

- Canning jars. Storing whole foods needs some special attention so it keeps well and doesn't attract pests.

- Stainless steel cookware. I had some deteriorating nonstick pans and I didn't want to go to all this investment only to be putting toxins from the pans in my body.

- Juicer (masticating). I had done some green juice fasts in the past and really loved the 'restart' aspect of it along with the energy boost and noticeably clearer skin. I decided to add some interest to my diet and eventually replace supplements like DIM by incorporating green juices into my diet on a more regular basis.

- Vitamix. Okay, I admit, I'd been wanting a Vitamix for some time now and just needed one more good reason to buy one. I wanted to explore some more complex recipes to keep myself focused on the things I could have (like super smooth avocado pudding pies, and vegan cheeses).

- Honey and maple syrup. I already had a pretty good grip on keeping sugar out of my diet, so this wasn't really mentioned by my naturopath; however, I wanted to remove sugar products from my cupboard and have only raw local honey and maple syrup available for sweetening.

- Ginger and turmeric root. I wanted to eventually replace the supplements I was taking with the real thing.

- Whole prepared food store locations. Truth is, I have a hard time always cooking for myself. Sometimes I want immediate food without the preparation hassle. Not only did the coffee ladies there: Franki and Pam[18] wean me from my doppio con panna habit by offering decaff espresso with coconut milk (Starbucks wasn't doing that yet!), I could also walk up and get steamed veggies, rice, whole fruits and seeds for any meal of the day.

- Probiotic supplement.

So even though it is possible to get sufficient probiotics via fermented food, because I was cutting out all dairy and fermented drinks, the naturopath suggested I take probiotic supplements.

I learned it is important to buy probiotics from reputable distributors because how they are stored affects their potency. I talked with the Vital-10 representatives directly because one shipment I had come to my house, I missed and the bottle cooked in my mailbox for four days during a 90+ degree heatwave. They emphasized the importance of getting these from sources on their trusted list (none of which are

Amazon sellers, by the way). Poor storage practices *will* negatively affect the probiotic quality, not so much the mailing.

Supplements

Besides conscious eating, the naturopath did suggest some supplements to help me get back into balance. All were intended to be taken for limited durations, except the probiotics and vitamin D which I take continuously, to this day.

In all cases I used the reputable brands my naturopath suggested.

The naturopath put select supplements together in 'rounds' and every month or so switched up the mix. I am not going to pretend to know the best things to combine at what strength for the best duration, so I did not list any below. You will need to reach out to a licensed naturopath you trust, and together identify what is best for you. Below is a list of supplements I used at one time or another during my healing experiment.

- Vitamin D
- DIM[19] (Diindolylmethane)
- L-5-MTHF (methyltetrahydrofolate)—the active form of folic acid
- Vitamin A
- Vitamin C[20]
- Oregano oil
- Ginger oil
- EGCg (green tea extract)
- Curcumin (turmeric)

As a guideline, I could tell my naturopath was recommending supplements based on her patients experience and results with using them. I did not let that stop me from researching them myself and pushing back on ones I didn't feel comfortable with. I was pleased to find posted studies associated with how these supplements improve the chances of regression of HPV and cervical dysplasia. I do have to mention, finding postings on the internet I considered to be of some reputable value was a challenge as there are so many people marketing these things. I encourage you to do your own research, the notes and references provide a good start.

A few worthy supplement study callouts:

- L-5-MTHF: "Insufficient intake of folate is associated with increased risk for cervical dysplasia." A lot of people have been looking into this! Here are a few: Liu 1993; Kwanbunjan 2004; Buckley 1992; Grio 1993; Kwasniewska 1997; Weinstein 2001; Butterworth 1992; Ziegler 1986; Hernandez 2003; Goodman 2001.

- Vitamin A: "Retinoids, the natural and synthetic forms of vitamin A, inhibit the growth of epithelial cells through transforming growth factor beta (Comerci 1997). Additionally, retinoids have been reported to support the differentiation of cells (thereby preventing abnormal cervical cancer cells), as well as to affect the immune response of cells" (Ahn 1997; Darwiche 1994).

- Green tea: "Green tea extracts in the form of a vaginal delivery and an oral capsule are effective strategies for treating cervical lesions."[21]

- Turmeric: "With regard to cervical cancer, turmeric affects the transcription of the high-risk variant HPV18 as well as other cellular transcription responses" (Prusty 2005).

Sensitivities

Like with your Western doctor, what is prescribed is just a well-educated guess that the drug will work for you.

Just because it says 'all natural' doesn't
mean it can't hurt you.
Be diligent.
Before you put anything into your
body, ask all your questions.
Do your best researching the supplement and its use.
Make sure you feel confident it will
contribute to your healing.

As an example, here are some unusual reactions I experienced.

- Vitamin C—generally people can tell when they are taking too much of it because they get diarrhea. I was taking a very large dose of vitamin C four times a day and still would continue to be constipated. My naturopath concluded my body just didn't pay much attention to this supplement, so I stopped taking it, ever. This experience has saved me some money by no longer buying vitamin-enhanced water and similar packaged powders.

- EGCg—I was taking this in a capsule instead of drinking ten cups of green tea a day. I did not get the jitters, I did not lose weight, so this again seemed to be kind of a nothing to my body. When I took these vaginally, I swelled up like crazy, so even though most everyone can take these, they are simply not of any good to me and I stopped taking it vaginally and orally. I also stopped buying and drinking green tea in general.

- Curcumin—this is generally taken by people on a daily basis as an inflammation control supplement. Turns out this gives me diarrhea, even in the form of a simple commercial turmeric tea. So even though most everyone can take this without any problem, it's not great for me. I typically only use it as a nice curry seasoning on my foods, and on occasion I add a small bit of the root to spice up my green juice.

Procedure for daily supplement management

I had never taken many pills before, so it was shockingly hard for me to organize how to take all the daily supplements. I was not only forgetting to take them, but I couldn't always remember when I did take them. Having a pill organizer was a must for me. On Sunday nights, I put together the week's worth of supplements.

Procedure

- Daily pill organizer (am/pm—big, detachable compartments). Since I didn't want to carry a big pallet of a week's worth of pills to my work or on short overnight travel, the detachable compartments worked out great.
- Medication reminder. Since I was taking some supplements four times a day, a reminder alarm was helpful.
- Medication list and provider synch. Since I was working with several doctors in different offices, I put effort into making sure they all knew about each other and everything I was putting into my body. It is unfortunate that there was no smart phone app or other data integration methods that could synchronize their data on me! Many of the supplements were

'unknown' to my Western primary provider's drug database. To my gyn's credit, he took the time during our visits to ask questions about some of the supplements and my thought process around deciding to pay for and take them. He also took time to help me discern good vs. crappy sites on the internet.

Vaginal suppository

The typical term for this treatment is vaginal suppositories. However, this was a frequent conversation between me and my partner, so we reduced a few syllables and called it the 'pussy pills'. When I was in company where saying 'pussy' didn't seem quite right, I called them 'unsavories'. Awkward words aside, the approach is to have a local treatment applied directly to the cervix to essentially remove the cell layer that is causing the problem.

Turns out there are many kinds of treatments that can accomplish this. The trick is finding the one that your body responds to the best. And for me, there were several rounds of trial and error.

There is a naturopathic treatment called Escharotic. This chemically dissolves the top layer of cells on the cervix. Truth is, I saw too many chemical burns gone bad on the internet to be comfortable with this. My naturopath dismissed it immediately as too harsh.

She suggested her go-to suppository 'cocktail' she had seen good results with. She combined the ingredients of a traditional vaginal depletion pack[22] with green tea and a soothing agent. The ingredients were all formed into a bullet-shaped suppository, and you put one up onto your vagina as close to the cervix as possible most every night. The initial optimistic duration of treatment was for five months.

Compounding Pharmacy

I had to go to a specific compounding pharmacy in town to pick up the custom-designed pussy pills. I had never heard of, nor been to a compounding pharmacy. To be clear, this isn't Walgreen's drive-through or Kaiser Pharmacy take-a-number by a long shot. The doctor had to call in the prescription seven days in advance of pick-up. The hours of operations were 9-12 am and 1-4 pm Monday through Thursday, so I had to take some time off work to go there. There was no storefront. I showed up to the address that was one of those 1980s two-story buildings in a business park. I went into the plain wooden door with the address number on it. Once inside there was about two feet of space to stand in front of a small walled-in pick-up window. I was the only customer there (or that could fit) and just kind of stood there wondering if anything in that suppository was from the black market. A person came to the window and asked me my name, then came back with a medium-sized foiled envelope. No drug description label. No little white bag. No ID checking. I paid on my credit card. That was it. I was a little dumbfounded and walked out with my foiled package like I just participated in some kind of secret drug drop.

Sometime later when picking up cervix gel, it was given to me in a little white lace gift bag.

It's not pretty

I understand that everyone's response to this treatment is unique to the individual; but 'stimulate the body to slough off abnormal cervical cells, and promote lymphatic drainage' *gets real.*

Me: (thanking God my naturopath answers emails) I have some questions on what is a 'normal' response to the suppository. I am having a mild burning sensation at night and then black fluid and white and black bits are coming out of me that looks like the stuff you scrap off when you re-caulk tiles in the bathroom.

Naturopath: That all sounds within the realm of normal. If the discomfort isn't ruining your day, keep it up.

So it's like that.

Materials list for vaginal suppositories

- Suppositories based on components in traditional vaginal depletion packs (with Thuja).
- Green tea suppositories.
- Vaginal suppositories for sensitive and irritated tissues.
- Gowey Gel (made from the pitcher plant).
- Boric Acid capsules. As aside worth mentioning: Boric acid can be used to treat bacterial vaginosis (BV). Not to be used *in combination* with the other vaginal treatments for cervical dysplasia, but it has never let me down in chasing away the occasional bout of BV or yeast infection.

Make it through vaginal suppositories feeling like a human

With all this going on down there, it was difficult for me to feel 'confident as a woman'. For me that woman confidence comes from feeling clean, sexy, healthy and strong.

Procedure for feeling clean

- Bidet appliance. I am not kidding, this is a life saver. This is basically a fancy toilet seat. They are available at all price ranges. I got one that warms the water and has a remote control. I like it so much I got one for my dad on Father's Day.

- Nightly shower. Yes, you will take another in the morning, so what? Treat yourself to the warm calm of a nightly shower. Rinse away what your body used and sloughed off during the day and prepare yourself for a fresh round of nightly healing.

- Cotton panties (motivational). If you are not used to sleeping in panties, you will want to while taking vaginal suppositories. So yes, your panties are going to get messy at night, it's what that pussy pill is supposed to do, after all. So instead of thinking of 'granny panties' I recommend a style and print that reminds you of how strong you are for facing this! I got Wonder Woman hipsters.

- Panty liners (organic cotton). After some research, I recommend organic cotton.

Keep a healthy sex life

Though I was already happy with my sex life, this gave me an opportunity to up my intimacy and trust game even more. Wait, what? Better sex with HPV? Well, I wouldn't go that far, but we definitely improved intimacy and trust.

Sex is a part of keeping my mind and spirit happy. Sex is certainly part of keeping joy in my life and an essential component in my healing experiment. For me, it was not only important to continue having a healthy sex life with my primary partner, it was important to keep him safe and my metamours (my partner's partner and their partners) safe.

Avoid additional HPV exposure

If you are having intimate interactions with another person where genitals may be in contact with your skin (any skin, mouth included), insist upon disclosing *anything* known about STI screenings, *including* high-risk HPV. Avoiding additional exposure to HPV, including additional strains you might not have yet, improves your chances of cervical dysplasia regression.

> When mutual respect and love is present,
> this conversation becomes a natural
> contribution to the relationship.

Maybe the relationship isn't that involved? Right? If there is hesitancy to have a detailed conversation about mutual respect, health and safety, I suggest that's probably a good indicator this person is not someone to be having an intimate activity with. If it's a 'fun night out' and nothing more, plan your sexual consent with this in mind: simply assume the person has every STI in the book and perhaps just doesn't know about it yet. Take a moment and try that on.

Maybe just yesterday you were that person.

Being tired is okay

I was sure to keep my partner in the know about how I was feeling—the physical and the mental details. While taking the anti-viral supplements and the vaginal suppositories I was very tired. My body and mind were directing a lot of energy to healing. That means our date nights shifted in hours and location. Sometimes we just showered and snuggled while watching Netflix. Sometimes we just snuggled and he kissed my forehead until I fell asleep.

> What's important is feeling physically
> and emotionally connected.

Sensation Play

This is the perfect time to explore feeling great in new ways. After going through all the testing and vaginal treatments, it makes sense that you may need to make a little extra space to gently and gradually ease back into sex. Feel the freedom to reduce or completely remove the focus from penetration. There are plenty of opportunities for creativity here to explore all parts of the body with all kinds of things. Wire head massager, plastic bendy drumming sticks of various kinds to drum your back or legs, back scratchers or other scratching devices, maybe even make claws of your fingers. Paddles, feathers, ice, hair, showers, etc. You get the idea.

Try out new sensations on all your senses: seeing new images or not seeing, allowing yourself to be seen. Hearing various sounds or not hearing, making sounds, allowing yourself to be heard or allowing yourself to be quieted. Tasting new tastes or not tasting.

Some may consider these explorations to be part of BDSM[23] play, but you certainly don't have to be a sadomasochist or interested in power dynamics to try things out. Let go of any preconceived notions and allow yourself to explore what uniquely feels good to you. Feeling good doesn't necessarily have to mean feeling excited, it can mean feeling calm and relaxed. You define for yourself what feeling good is and do that!

This not only relieves any fear or discomfort you may be having, but it can help to regain a sense of security about your body. Allow yourself to be in the moment, breathe in the joy. Feel gratitude for your amazing body and for your partner's generosity.

What's important is feeling delight in your body.

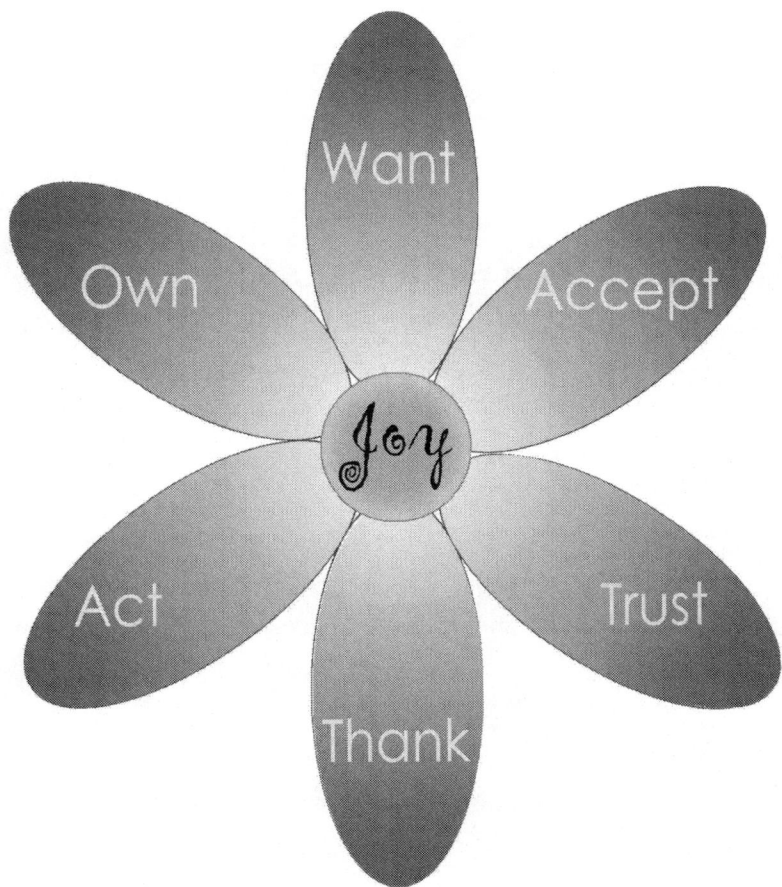

Materials list for a healthy sex life while using pussy pills

- Consent. Take the time for open and honest conversation. Ensure you and your partner are 100% on the same page. For me and my primary partner, the term "tonight is a pussy pill night" was an important starter to our agreements around how we would approach physical intimacy that day.

- Oxytocin. The daily dose of oxytocin as it naturally occurs from having sex is as important as the daily supplements! You may want to investigate the effects of oxytocin on the female body.[24]

- Sensory exploration objects. Be creative!

- Sanitize-able toys (i.e. silicone or glass). Only use objects that are sanitize-able on your genitals. You don't want to be counterproductive by introducing the virus again and again. HPV-16 can still be infective even after being dehydrated on a surface for 7 days.[25] Always use only your toys only on you, and boil them between use.

- Condoms (non-latex). The components of the suppositories may not react well with latex, so non-latex condoms are a must. After some trial and error, I found these seem to run small. If your partner typically counts on the stretchy nature of the typical latex condom to get them on and be comfortable, get the 'magnum' size.

- Lubricant (water-based with carrageenan). The suppository has a significant drying effect, so always use lubricant with anything you insert into your vagina or rectum. Carrageenan inhibits HPV 16.[26]

- Towels. You can relax and enjoy yourself more knowing anything messy is going to get sopped up on an easy to clean towel.

Letting go

There were a few things I had to give up because they just don't go with trying to heal cervical skin. The naturopath suggested limited hot tub time and swimming (no more than once a week). I just didn't feel comfortable biking anymore. My 'letting go' list, beyond food habits, was, in truth, short.

Trial and error

After my first round of the vagi-pak/green tea combo suppository for five months, I stopped using it for a month to let my cervix and vagina 'rest' and then went in for a follow-up Pap. The labs came back the same. No change. This result was disappointing, to say the least.

For Round 2 we tried the same vaginal suppositories plus added straight up green tea capsules vaginally. This mini-experiment was very enlightening. Within just a few days of this, my vagina swelled up significantly, almost entirely, so that even with lubricant I could not fit in a capsule (or my finger). So, even though it is very rare, my body was essentially allergic to green tea, which I was giving it consistently this whole time. So now we knew to remove green tea from my treatment plan.

Round 3 was suppositories designed for sensitive, irritated tissues that included calendula. Time for another Pap, and still no change.

I admit, my resolve was starting to waver. Though I was a little weary, I was still clinically in a position to regress. So I was ready for the next recommendation. This time was different: no more suppositories, now cervical gel made from a pitcher plant. This treatment is branded The Gowey Protocol.[27] The doctor who developed this gel has several videos; my favorite is when she says "Don't freak out yet, there are still things you can do to get yourself healthy".[28] She also has a book titled "Your Cervix Just has a Cold".

The naturopath painted my cervix with the gel once a month and every night I applied some myself with an injector applicator. And finally, with the next Pap there was an improvement. My healing was finally measurable. It took several more rounds of the gel, but in the end there were no more abnormal cells, and no more HPV.

Yep. There it is, no more abnormal cells and no more HPV.

I still remember that moment when I let that sink in. I was in my car taking a break from a festival and checking my phone for messages. It was hot and the car had that sitting-in-an-oven feeling that is really delicious for about the first minute or two. And there was the email that my test results were in. I read it several times and had to cry a little. The rest of the day was a bit of a blissful fog.

Like any major transformation there were a lot of changes in progress at the same time, but on this front, the letting go of the abnormal cervical cells finally occurred. The pitcher plant was my most valuable player.

The other important front: the battle of the mind.

Visualize your cervix as a healthy pink donut.
—Dr. Brandie Gowey, NMD

Procedure 2: Yoga practice

When I started the allergy elimination diet and the first round of the vaginal suppositories, I didn't really take the yoga part that seriously. Yes, I continued to attend a weekly class, and yes, I did learn a couple of breathing techniques which I performed during class. But, honestly, that was about it. Oh, remember that pose I wanted to master by my next screening? The freak-out conversation I had with my yoga teacher where she instructed me to breathe? Well, that "ten weeks to accomplishing the eight-angle pose" had come and gone, and my progress in the pose was no more than learning the warm-up sequence. I admit I wasn't feeling committed in the beginning.

Joy will propel you forward

I had good friend/co-worker who took me to the occasional happy hour on a consistent basis for several years. He always let me pick where were went. We tried all kinds of things: hip places with jazzy drinkologists, beer at the pizza pub, snooty wine bars, whatever came with tater tots across the street from work, trendy micro-brewery, and if a cupcake place was nearby that was a bonus. We laughed, debriefed work, shared funny stories, yeah, it was a joy. During this time when he asked to schedule our next after-work drink, I picked out a Mediterranean grocery store that had not only a wine bar, but also a juice bar. When I ordered a green juice instead of my typical martini, I knew that move was the opening to a conversation unlike our typical workplace debriefing.

Friend: Okay, what's up with the weird green juice order?

Me: Yeah, well, you know that martini we had last time in the Rainbow Room (my favorite martini bar, server was always beautifully dressed in drag and she made the best vanilla martini in town handsdown)? Well, that may have been my last martini.

Friend: What? Really? Why?

Me: (gulping a bit, recognizing this was a moment to stick with my decision to have an open conversation that breaks all needless shame barriers) Well, I have stage-zero cervical cancer, and alcohol doesn't mix with my treatments. (Okay, good, close enough to what's going on, and all said in one short sentence, did it!) I am not really telling people at work though (just to be sure).

Friend: (because he's a real friend, he made me say a little more) Okay. So, how are you feeling?

Me: (wanting to share something significantly honest, but none of the gory details of the pussy pills which was a constant discomfort) It's the head game, that's what's hard, it's exhausting. I am always so tired.

And there it was. Through no effort of his own, just by being who he is, my friend helped me acknowledge what I needed to face next. It was clear I needed to face my racing mind. I already had one measurement show no positive progress and this was putting me into a downward spiral.

I needed something more to turn this around. I knew I was ready for the mind training.

Winning the head-game

It just so turned out, my yoga teacher was offering a brand new online training. It lasted 108 days. She said, no matter what you choose to focus on, you do it consistently for 108 days and that will make a significant difference. This was it! I signed up during the early-bird period.

* * *

Naming a change I wanted to see in myself was straightforward: I wanted that next Pap test to be negative. How I got there via the yoga wasn't really a concern of mine; I would completely trust my teacher on that. She already mentioned breathing was important, so I would use that as my place to focus.

What she prescribed as the practice was also very simple: walk the walk every day, for 108 days.

Waking up

Interestingly enough, to do a daily yoga practice, you actually have to get out of bed. For me, a lifelong snooze button addict, this was a serious challenge. For the first week of my 108-day daily yoga practice I committed only to this: when the alarm went off, I would flop myself out of bed, sit quietly and drink a cup of herbal tea.

Yep. That's it. This was surprisingly difficult for me and an important ground zero procedure. I have been waking up my entire life—getting the kids ready for daycare and school, getting me ready for work. Honestly, I thought I was a pro at it.

> This was different. This was waking up to be peaceful and joyful: Not waking to rush into the day, but waking to train my mind.

As I struggled with this change, I noticed that what made it difficult for me was the dark and the cold that met me outside of the covers. I didn't want that to get in my way so I got a few luxury items to help along the transition to starting my day with warmth.

Materials list for waking up

- Sunrise alarm clock (with wake-up light and nature sounds)
- Lemon water
- Organic herbal tea (chai, ginger and turmeric)
- Electric boiler (with timer)
- Sitting shawl (natural fiber)
- Warm socks.
- Space heater (with timer and oscillation)
- Meditation cushion (firm and elevating)
- Mantra ("Om Gam Ganapataye Namaha")

Pawanmuktasana Series 1

If you're looking topics up on the internet as you read along, there is a very beneficial pose that is spelled very much the same as this—pavanamuktasana: the 'wind relieving pose'. Though that's a fantastic position, it is *not* the procedure I am referencing here in my healing experiment.

To read the full description of the Pawanmuktasana Series you can reference the incredibly comprehensive illustrated yoga manual, "Asana Pranayama Mudra Bandha." Pawanmuktasana is described as "a group of asanas that remove any blockages which prevent the free flow of energy in the body and mind."[29] My yoga teacher taught me to do a practice that is similarly described in the Pawanmuktasana

Series Part 1 of this book, with the movements done with synchronized breathing and prana awareness breaks. She added a breathing exercise at the end that involves inhaling fully and holding the breath in and sipping it in even further until finally it's necessary to fully exhale.

I am by no means qualified nor capable to teach this practice in my experimental healing procedure, no more than I am able to prescribe herbal remedies previously described in the naturopathic procedure. If you are interested in trying out this yoga practice, please connect with a qualified hatha yoga instructor. That said, you can get an idea about what this is by searching videos on the internet. I have yet to find a free video that demonstrates the integrated breathing as I was taught; you might want to look into online subscription offerings.

Preparation

As preparation for morning practice, I chose to try and train myself to poop every day upon waking. Now the first time this was suggested to me, I giggled to myself at how unrealistic that is. All my adult life I could only count on pooping about every other day, and pooping on command was only something I had trained my Doberman to do! That said, daily pooping was also on my naturopath's set of things to strive for in gut health, so I decided to give it an honest try. The Ayurvedic position of pooping is squatting, with your thighs pressing into your belly, and then you relax, exhale and suck your belly button in and up. This also seemed very impossible to me. There was no position I could get into where my thighs touched my abdomen and balancing on my toilet was just not going to happen: yes, I did try, failed and laughed very loudly! At that point, I didn't even get to try the notion of sucking in my belly button. What I was successful in was getting a squatting toilet stool and consistently using it.

Another, much easier preparation for morning practice is the commitment to tongue scraping. The idea of removing that morning mucus coating off my tongue just sounded right, and I had been brushing my tongue my whole life; this just sounded more thorough. And if it did 'promote overall digestive health,' that was just a great bonus in my mind.

So as soon as I learned Pawanmuktasana, I incorporated it into my daily waking up practice. I spent less time waking up and drinking tea so I had time to move and breathe through this series. As my own choice, typically I did a full version of this on the weekends (20-30 minutes) and a shortened version of it (5-10 minutes) during the working week days.

For me the synchronized breathing in and out my nose made for the release of snot! Both through my nose and by causing me to cough. This is all good according to my teacher, and you can tell it's good, because it feels good. However, I find it helpful to keep a tissue nearby.

Though a yoga mat isn't really necessary, for this practice, I decided to get a new all-natural mat (and let my old chemical-based one hold my hallway rug down). After some research, I ended up getting a rubber mat; however, some people are sensitive to this material. It's worth mentioning that the smell of a new rubber mat can be overwhelming. Be sure in the first few days of use to wipe it down well with vinegar water spray and hang it to air it out instead of just immediately rolling it up after use.

This practice is designed for anyone; young or old, healthy or sick, physically strong or weak. It doesn't matter. It is all done in a seated position. So even when (especially when) I wasn't feeling well, I still did this practice. I could feel the benefit of it immediately and accumulatively. It was easy to notice that this made a positive difference in how my day started. Overall, this practice brought about a profound change in my life: if you choose to do only one yoga practice, I recommend this one.

Materials list for Pawanmuktasana

- Qualified Hatha yoga instructor
- Squatty potty
- Tongue scraper (metal)
- All natural yoga mat (rubber)
- Box of tissues

Mantra: instrument of thought

Mantra was a complete surprise to me, in that it apparently is the essence of mind training. Developed before language, sources do not agree on what mantra is. I follow the thinking of my yoga instructor, that it is a prayer and divine vibration. There are many mantra ranging from a single syllable to long phrases.

I chose to pick just one to focus on, the Ganesh mantra, "Om Gam Ganapataye Namaha." I chose this mantra because I love the image of an elephant-headed deity removing obstacles for me! By choosing to chant this I feel the virus, the abnormal cells, the stigma, all those things I am ready to let go of just being completely removed from my thinking, my body and my life. It honestly makes me giggle a bit, and I like that part! For me, mantra easily replaces worrying thoughts with inspiration.

As soon as I learned the Ganesh mantra, I incorporated it into my daily waking up practice. I found a song version of this on YouTube that I enjoy, and play it while I do my bathroom asana preparation time. It repeats 108 times and takes about six minutes to go through. It is not advised that you multi-task with mantra. However, I find it comforting to chant as a 'background' activity and especially enjoy chanting it while I am in the shower.

Gratitude

At the end of each morning practice, I take moment to thank—just whatever thanking that seemed to arise. I thank my yoga teacher for giving me these tools and procedures for my healing experiment, I thank the other yoga students in the 108-day course for being there with me, I thank Ganesh for taking away my obstacles, some days I thank the bacteria for being balanced in their occupation of my body, the cells in my body for growing in a healthy way, my immune system for always knowing exactly what to do, heck I thank the viruses for leaving!

Every day it was something new and different to be grateful for. Soon, I found it a bit surprising that in my meditation I was thanking those people who healed me; it felt like my being healed had already happened. *And that was the turning point.*

> When I felt as though there was no longer any reason to worry about my healing. I knew I had won the head game.

Procedure of my daily practice

When all the steps of my new daily yoga practice came together, it looked like this:

1. Get out of bed.
2. Space heater on to warm my yoga mat.
3. Drink a cup of warm lemon water (electric pot already had my water hot).

4. Listen and sing along with the Ganesh mantra. (6 minutes)

5. Poop using squatty potty and bidet.

6. Brush my teeth and scrape my tongue.

7. Sit on my meditation cushion with my cozy shawl and finish my tea and mantra.

8. Do Pawanmuktasana with breath exercise. (5-20 minutes)

9. Savor a moment of gratitude.

It wasn't hard to notice the immediate and continuous expansion of peace of mind, my sense of self-acceptance and my feeling of general wellness. And then, my vision of gratitude expanded, into something so significant, it became a key component in my healing experiment.

Procedure 3: Thank-you

Early in my healing experiment, during my nightly internet searches, I decided to order some books on the topic. One title that caught my eye was "Thank You for HPV," by Zayna De Gaia.

My gut response to that? What kind of hippy, sunshine, bologna is this? If I was talking to HPV it would sound a bit more sarcastic, like "HPV: Thanks for Nothing." Yes, intellectually I understood about the life learning and awareness thing, but deep down I sure didn't feel thankful for this situation. Right there in the middle of uncomfortable treatments and many lifestyle changes, I was not feeling particularly grateful.

I didn't really think about gratitude as being *part of* my healing until I noticed I was spending more and more of my meditation time running dialogues in my mind thanking people. Not only could I hear my voice thanking them, I could hear their responses.

Then I became a bit obsessed with planning how I was going to thank all these people. What would I say? Should I give them a thank-you note? A small gift?

Where were these thoughts coming from? Maybe this was due to the long, consistent (often annoying and painful) training of my grandma and mother forcing me to write and deliver thank-you cards all though my growing up. Or maybe it was when I was a real estate broker, and there was pressure to have very hip closing gifts. The reason didn't really matter; the visions kept forming, there was no stopping them.

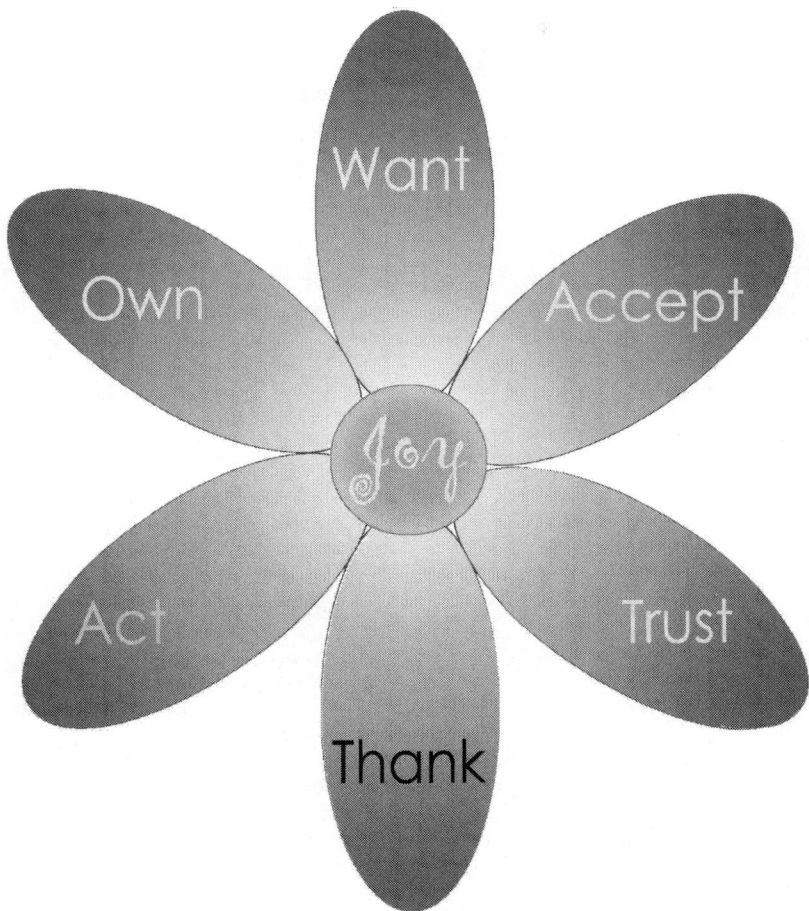

Want

Own

Accept

Joy

Act

Trust

Thank

A vision of gratitude

I have a nice succulent arrangement in my living room—given to me a year ago by my co-workers when my brother died. I love that plant; not only because it was one of the few plants that was thriving in my house, but because it made me smile when I looked at it. During those moments I remembered my brother and my co-workers' thoughtfulness.

From this feeling, a vision of gratitude sprouted—I envisioned myself bringing a living plant to my naturopath's office. I wanted the whole office to know I appreciated them. I wanted to give something everyone could enjoy that would last a long time (like my series of office visits!).

I found myself visiting nurseries during my lunch hour to find similar arrangements and where a wide selection of succulents were readily available. Those trips to the nursery were the beginning of my making my visions of wellness and gratitude become my reality.

I had a small friendship coin that my girlfriend gave me a couple years ago when we were on one of our "girlfriend trips." When I ran across it in my coin purse, it made me smile and think of my girlfriend's support and love. I liked the way I could carry it around with me easily, forget about it and then unexpectedly re-find it, rub it gently between my fingers, or squeeze it in my palm. I thought it was a bit magical how such a simple object could immediately make me feel so close to my best friends.

From this feeling, more visions of gratitude formed—I wanted to give this feeling to the people who were helping me heal. I started browsing the internet for small similar coins that said 'thank you' or 'gratitude' on them. I kept my thank-you coin stash (smiling suns in cute little yellow gift bags) on top of my dresser in a tray near my meditation candle and incense burner. I was saving them: for *that* moment, when I got that first negative lab result that proved I was truly healed. That's when I would deliver them.

> I realized every time I visited a nursery or saw those coins on my dresser, I felt healed. Feeling gratitude started to equate to feeling healed.

Motivation

My visions of gratitude came to me consistently during my morning meditation. The joyful feeling it brought me was undeniable and slightly addictive! I noticed that the intention behind my wanting to extend thanks wasn't like other moments of saying thank-you that I'd had before. It isn't to differentiate myself amongst others. It's not about demonstrating my creativity or uniqueness. It's not to spotlight one of my thank-ees over the other. It's not to grow my 'account' with my healers. It's not about retaining these people as my friends.

I admit, however, this is just as self-serving as those reasons. This helped me have so much belief and faith in my healing that I could already feel what it's like to be transformed. I could truly think of myself as healthy. Right now.

> You don't have to wait for something wonderful to happen to be thankful for it. Create a vision of gratitude and feel thankful for having what you want right now.

Thank people who don't know they are healing you

My co-workers had no idea I was working through this issue. I always kept my medical conditions private at the workplace—I just didn't want to be one of *those* people, who expect some kind of special treatment—like we didn't all have life circumstances to deal with.

I began to imagine an announcement to my co-workers at a team meeting. During this announcement, I would pass around the small tray of gratitude coins so that each person could take one if they wanted to. That's it. Pretty simple vision of gratitude.

I imagined this every day—looking at the coins on my dresser reminded me. I imagined the meeting room, the donuts, their faces, their distraction with their laptops, people fidgeting with their chairs and each person's unique postures, the projector on with the agenda presented, the smell of the carpet, the glow of the fluorescent lights, everything. When I was in real life having a team meeting at work, I would daydream about this agenda item.

In this announcement, I would tell them they were unknowingly part of my healing just by being in my vision of gratitude—and I would thank them for that. It didn't matter to me if they could even understand what I was describing.

When it isn't a vision anymore, it's my real life

I admit, on the real-life day I arranged for this long-anticipated event as an agenda item in our team meeting, I seriously considered backing out. After all, I already regressed. The dysplasia was healed, the HPV resolved. I really didn't have to tell them anything. They didn't know anything before, they didn't really need to know anything now. Some of the staff didn't even know me most of the time I was working through all this. The whole thing kind of sounded crazy to me at this point, so I was sure it would sound crazy to them too.

But, I felt somehow, I would be cheating the universe if I didn't go through with it.

When I was contemplating whether it was 'worth it' to go through with the plan to distribute the gratitude coins, I figured—when it came right down to it—I wanted to remind them of how precious they are. Just the way they are, with no specific effort of their own, they are healing others and that they healed me.

For all I knew, by my going through with enacting this vision I could be part of someone else's healing—right?

So with a shaky voice and a few tears, I did what I imagined for so long.

> And then, for one full breathless moment—
> everyone just loved each other.

It was one of the most profound moments of my life.

I realized, I created a future moment. When you really think about it, we do that all the time. But here it was, so undeniably true: the thank-you procedure was envisioned, planned, conducted, measured—verified.

Thank yourself frequently

I was, after all, the star of the show in this. I decided to trust myself. I decided to trust my body and mind to heal itself. I based my healing procedures not only around the advice of my alternative medicine coaches, but at the root, on my own capabilities. The things my body and mind do without me even thinking about it are amazing!

During my meditation time, I thanked myself—every day. A frequent point of gratitude was thanking all my cells and the bacteria that lived with them, for working so hard in achieving a balance that made me healthy. Yeah, it's like that. And much more.

Materials list for thank-you

- A thoughtful message

- A token, can be touched and easily carried (gratitude coins)

- Visual display, can be seen frequently or shared by many people (potted plant)

- A symbol of a personal connection or shared experience (incense holder)

- Wrapping to show value in the act of giving (organza fabric bags)

Measurement: Cervical cancer screenings

Consistently measuring the progress of my healing was important to me for two reasons:

1. If the HPV and abnormal cells were *the same or going away*, I didn't want any emotions, worry, or the influence of other people's concerns to take over and drive me to capitulate to unnecessary treatments. I wanted to know if I was still in the situation where my body could heal itself, so I could stay out of its way and let it continue its excellent work in taking care of me.

2. If the HPV and abnormal cells were *progressing toward cancer* to the point where there was no longer a known chance of a full regression, I wanted to be in a position to begin mainstream treatment protocols as immediately as possible.

It's that simple. Only the established screenings could verify my hypothesis that my body would heal itself given the chance.

I didn't have to be creative to know how long to wait between measurements since the American Congress of Obstetricians and Gynecologists (ACOG) already did the work to establish an informed schedule for Well-Woman ages 40-64 and Cervical Cancer Screening ages 30-65.

So, I went in every three months (twelve weeks) for a follow-up Pap with HPV lab testing. Besides the emotional toll, it takes time and money to continuously go in for these. These repeat visits get, well, depressing.

That said, it was absolutely necessary to my healing experiment to have measurement guidelines, and not just because that was how I was going to validate my hypothesis; measurements are also an effective tool in helping stay the course and keep moving forward.

* * *

It's hard work to continue acting according to the plan, especially when thoughts that sound like voices keep creeping into the background and saying things like 'how can I just get this over with?' or 'can't I just quit caring about this?'

Re-energizing is absolutely necessary when the going gets tough.

That's where Joy comes in. It's in the center of the process for a reason!

PART 2

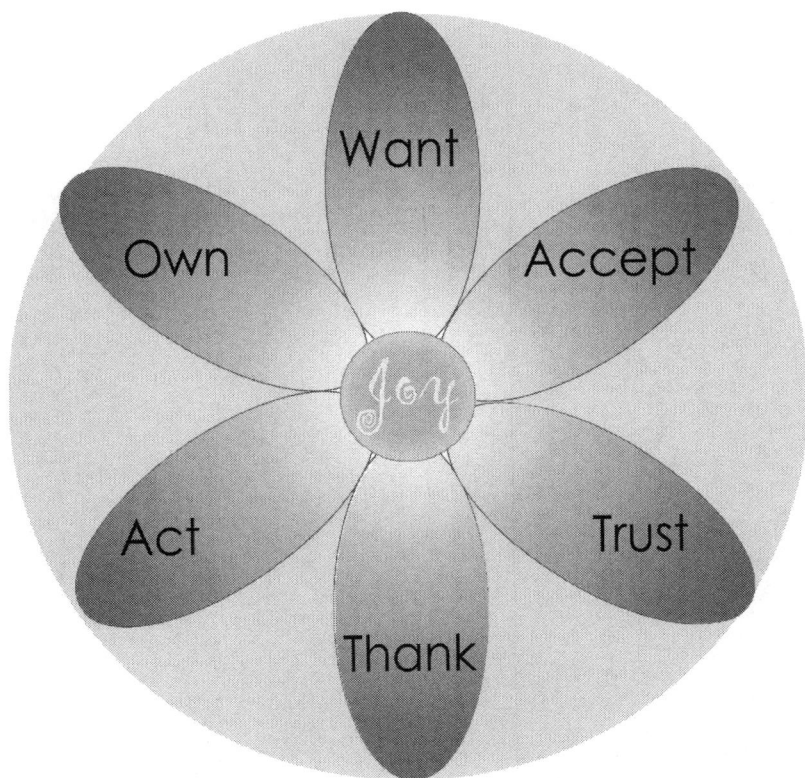

Your healing experiment—starts with Joy

In the next section of this book we walk through the decision-making process that will facilitate the development of your own healing experiment.

An essential foundation is knowing what your Joy is.

Once you can put words to your Joy, it's important to make the commitment to prioritize the placement of your Joy *in the middle of* your decisions and actions. Know that your Joy is going to be an oasis to go to when things get uncomfortable and the unexpected arises: you will need Joy to keep you going.

Notice the transformation model does *not* look like this.

It doesn't look like this either.

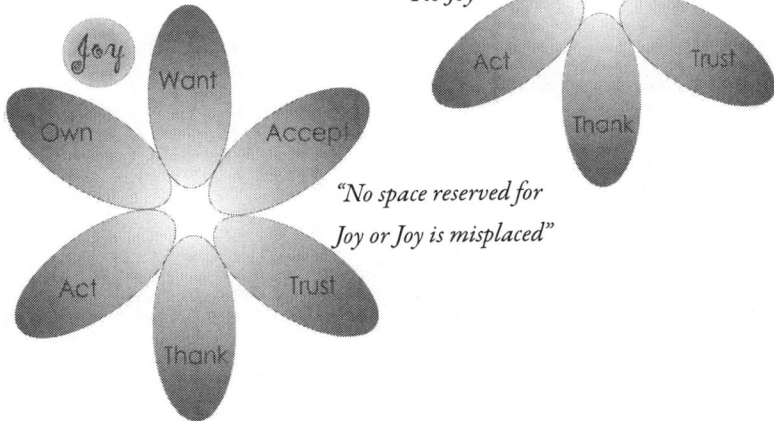

No Joy

"*No space reserved for Joy or Joy is misplaced*"

Joy will not help you through the tough times if there is no space for it in your decision-making or your life.

If Joy is just left out to bounce around in the areas where you always feel comfortable, or when you have time for it—the likelihood of getting the results you are hoping for are reduced. Besides, you might as well have some fun during your healing transformation journey!

Feeling Alive

Okay, so you are ready to define your Joy, but maybe it's just not really coming to you. After all, facing HPV and cervical dysplasia is not generally what people would consider fun at all, so how can I find things that make me feel good?

Consider this: What makes you feel really alive?

- Alive like, you can't wait to tell someone about it

- Alive like, you can't stop planning for it

- Alive like even when something goes sideways while you are doing it, that's just part of the fabulous adventure

- Alive like, you go to bed with that ridiculous smile on your face

- Maybe you even giggle a little to yourself when you think about it in the shower

I have a friend who shared with me a great example of someone who has found his Joy. He was a previous co-worker, and we get together every now and then to catch up on things. The last time I met him, as soon as we hugged hello, he immediately pulled out his phone.

Friend: (still riding the bliss wave, he could hardly contain himself) I have to show you this video. You know that raft I bought last year? Well I got one of those GoPros and strapped it to my helmet, and check this out! See that, yeah, every person in the raft in front of us was in the water. Then we all had to do a mini-rescue mission. With only one raft, several had to wait for us to come back and get them with the car. I stayed with the hurt guy. He was fine, just a little sore and shaken up. Do you believe that? I love that raft. I love being on the water.

Me: Wow, that's incredible. So, do you have more video of everyone still *in* the boat? You know, the actual rafting part?

Friend: No, not really, this happened just like minutes after we were a bit down river from the place where we put in.

Me: Oh my, so you only rafted just a few minutes and then helped the others the whole *rest* of your rafting day?

Friend: Yeah (chuckling to himself) it was still great. Rafting, all of it, it just makes me feel really alive. You know? I will take it any way I can get it!

Me: (to myself) Hey, I'm not judging what other people consider an 'alive' moment, but OMG does that sound like a crap day to me! And yet . . . there is no denying that smile I see on his face, the sparkle in his eye and the excitement in his voice.

Define your Joy

This is clearly not about what brings your friends Joy.

This is not about what you wish you want.

Not what your mom thinks brings Joy.

It's certainly not about what social media is currently selling as Joy.

> You can only find your Joy by looking within you.

The great part is you don't have to change anything, it's already there inside of you. It doesn't matter if what makes you feel alive is on the fringe of social acceptance. It's what matters to you, and having it in your life. The more you can feel it every day, the better; it will compel you to adopt new habits and activities.

> Within the context of your healing experiment, your Joy will be the catalyst for your procedures.

So now let's try and put some words to it around a few examples.

Finding Joy in I-just-know-what-I-know

You know when there are things you just will have, no matter what? Press into that and observe where your Joy is within that.

Example: I am not sure what it is, but when I am with her, I feel so alive.

My Joy is having her as my partner, she is worth fighting for.

- During the WANT step, this is a driver for choice-making. Envision how you will be with her as part of the solution, the place you will be in the end-game.

- In the ACCEPT step, think about how things are currently going between the two of you and if there is something you want to be sure to preserve or elevate.

- In the TRUST step, include her contribution to your desired outcome as defined in your hypothesis.

- In the THANK step, envision your gratitude for the feelings she gives you. Envision what you might say to her, or a small note or gift you might present to her.

- For the ACT step, include time and activities for being with her.

- When you OWN the outcome, she will be part of the ongoing care and feeding of your happiness and healthiness, perhaps in a way that 'pays it forward.'

Finding Joy in fear

Remember that freak-out moment? Those fears are actually pretty useful. Press into them and see where your Joy is within them.

Example: I am afraid of not having good health again. My joy is feeling strong and capable. My physical, mental and emotional well-being is worth fighting for.

- During the WANT step, this is a driver for choice-making. Envision what it looks like to be strong and capable with every decision and action.

- In the ACCEPT step, think about how you are currently feeling about your health, strength and wellbeing and if there is anything you need to lovingly accommodate or work around.

- In the TRUST step, trust in how your body and mind can heal themselves. Include your own body's healing capabilities to your desired outcome as defined by your hypothesis.

- In the THANK step, envision your gratitude for how truly amazing and awesome your body is in healing itself! It demonstrates this time after time, and remember, even *before* you see evidence of healing, envision your gratitude and the feelings you will have when you do.

- For the ACT step, plan into your healing procedures time and methods to notice your strength and capabilities.

- When you OWN the outcome, think about the ongoing care and feeding you may do to nurture your continued physical, mental and emotional strength and wellness. Think of your-self as healthy the same way you think of brushing your teeth in the morning. Consider what you might do to 'pay it for-ward' to someone else.

Finding Joy in what's been avoided, ignored, or put off

Remember that slap in the face feeling when you got the diagnosis? Is there some 'reality' about yourself that you've known about but have been covering up or hiding? Is there something you have always wanted to have or do but haven't made space for it in your life yet?

Now is the time to address these things—as Joy—in the center of your process.

- During the WANT step, these are a driver for your choices. Envision how your resolution to these things will be part of the solution.

- In the ACCEPT step, think about why you previously have been ignoring this and consider if there is something you want to let go of or do differently this time.

- In the TRUST step, include how facing these topics contrib-utes to your desired outcome as defined in your hypothesis.

- In the THANK step, envision your gratitude for the feelings you have knowing these topics are no longer outstanding.

- For the ACT step, include time and activities for fulfilling these outstanding issues.

- When you OWN the outcome, define what the ongoing care and feeding of these topics are, perhaps in a way that 'pays it forward' for others addressing the same or similar things.

Your Joy

Take a moment now to write down a few notes about your Joy.

What's Important

Being authentic, acknowledging your desires, your fears, what you seem to be avoiding. Describe those when you feel in the moment.

Brainstorm first—then go back and circle the ones that really resonate for you and use those to focus in on the following steps of the transformation process.

Things that make you feel alive

_____

_____

_____

_____

_____

_____

_____

_____

_____

_____

_____

_____

Joy building tips

- Make space to do those things that make you feel alive. Schedule them on your calendar if you need to.

- Take a break from a treatment cycle. I scheduled a cruise that fell in the middle of the cycle of a vaginal suppository round. "Take the week off" said the naturopath, and that sure put a big smile on my face!

- Trust your intuition (prove it to yourself by acting on it).

- Expand your vision of gratitude (observe how that changes your actions).

- Grow self-acceptance (observe the changes that brings about).

- Celebrate progress in your healing by looking for a chance to help someone.

- Acknowledge the feeling of bliss after meditation (anticipate that feeling for the next day).

- It is important to continue feeling joy while you are going through all this. If you tie your approach to each step to what makes you smile and feel bliss, you can feel joy every day of your treatment procedures.

You can always do retail therapy if you have room on your credit card.

—Drove a friend to LEEP,
then went shopping afterward

One process, infinite possibilities

In Part One, you read about how I applied the process I practiced thousands of times in my career to create my own healing experiment. Woven into that you've heard some other voices of experience based on women I interviewed that are just like you—like us!

In the last section you put into words notions of your own Joy, that you can count on to continuously propel you forward.

You are now fully equipped to go through the transformation process for yourself.

> At its core: it is a systematic approach to collecting observations and making decisions; a process to establish commitment.

These decisions don't have to happen in any given order and you don't have to have all the decisions made before you begin to act.

As a guide, we start at the top, and by the time we get through the third petal you will have enough information to create your healing hypothesis.

This diagram provides an overview of each step we will go through to create the hypothesis for, conduct, and verify the results of your own healing experiment.

Transformation Model
It's About Decision Making

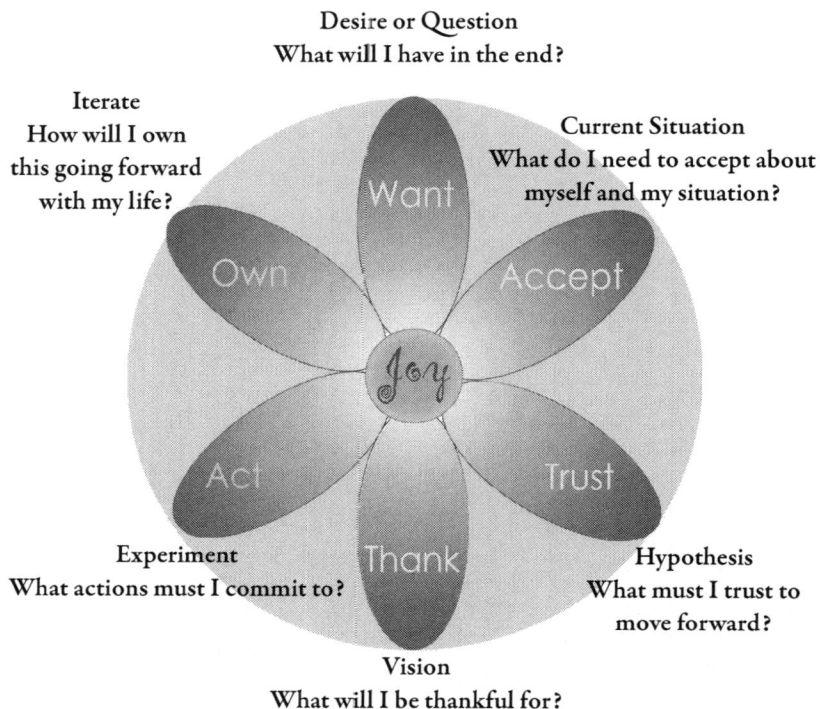

Desire or Question
What will I have in the end?

Iterate
How will I own
this going forward
with my life?

Current Situation
What do I need to accept about
myself and my situation?

Want

Own

Accept

Joy

Act

Trust

Experiment
What actions must I commit to?

Thank

Hypothesis
What must I trust to
move forward?

Vision
What will I be thankful for?

Observations become actionable decisions

Start at the top of the model and walk around it clockwise. Make a simple self-observation with each step:

1. What do I want in the end?

2. What do I need to accept about myself and my current situation?

3. What must I trust to move forward?

4. What will I be thankful for?

5. What actions must I commit to?

6. How will I own this going forward in my life?

Want

Question what you know *must* happen in the end. It's what you want so deeply, you just know it's going to happen. If possible, tie this to what gives you joy. When this is answered honestly, it guides your upcoming choices.

Decide what you want.

Accept

This is about acknowledging what is going on right now, inside of you and around you. Honest observation of your current circumstance will help you understand what will affect your ability to realistically move forward. After you decide what you will have, you also need to fully believe you can have it.

Decide what you believe.

Trust

You are ready to form your hypothesis. This requires reflection on your key decision and self-acceptance plus an initial round of research on who or what can help you with those things in mind. How are you going to go about validating your hypothesis?

Decide who and what you trust.

Thank

This is about planning. Begin to feel gratitude for your healing as soon as possible. Don't wait; describe who you will thank and how you will thank them *as part of* your experiment.

Decide on a vision you are willing to make reality.

Act

This is where you conduct your experiment (aka treatment plan): perform the procedures to prove out your hypothesis, prepare for delivering thank-you, and fill the experience with moments of joy.

Decide to commit.

Own

After you have drawn conclusions from your experiment's results, there is now something new in you that you will carry forward with you in your life. Reflect on you will do with what you have learned.

Decide to celebrate the change.

> Self-observation becomes decision,
> decision leads to action,
> action brings about transformation.

My example of the transformation process applied to my HPV/cervical dysplasia healing experiment

Want: I will have my whole cervix and my whole sex life. I will talk openly with those I love about my condition enabling me to discover and pursue everything I need to heal.

Accept: I accept my stubbornness, lifestyle choices and age: I embrace these aspects of myself as powerful contributions to my healing.

Trust: I trust that if I follow my naturopath's and yoga instructor's advice fully and consistently measure the progress of my healing, I will safely create the conditions my body needs to heal.

Thank: I thank my doctors, their staff, my family, instructors, and co-workers for providing me with their contribution to my healing. I will present them a small physical token they can hold or look at that can remind them of their positive impact just by being who they are.

Act: I will be true to my inner voice and commit to daily practices as prescribed by my naturopath and yoga instructor. I prioritize events on my/my partners' calendars that make me feel truly alive. I will consistently measure my progress by going to my Western gynecologist for follow-up screenings. I am planning and acquiring gratitude gifts.

Own: I will share tips and information I have learned with others, so they might have an opportunity for similar results.

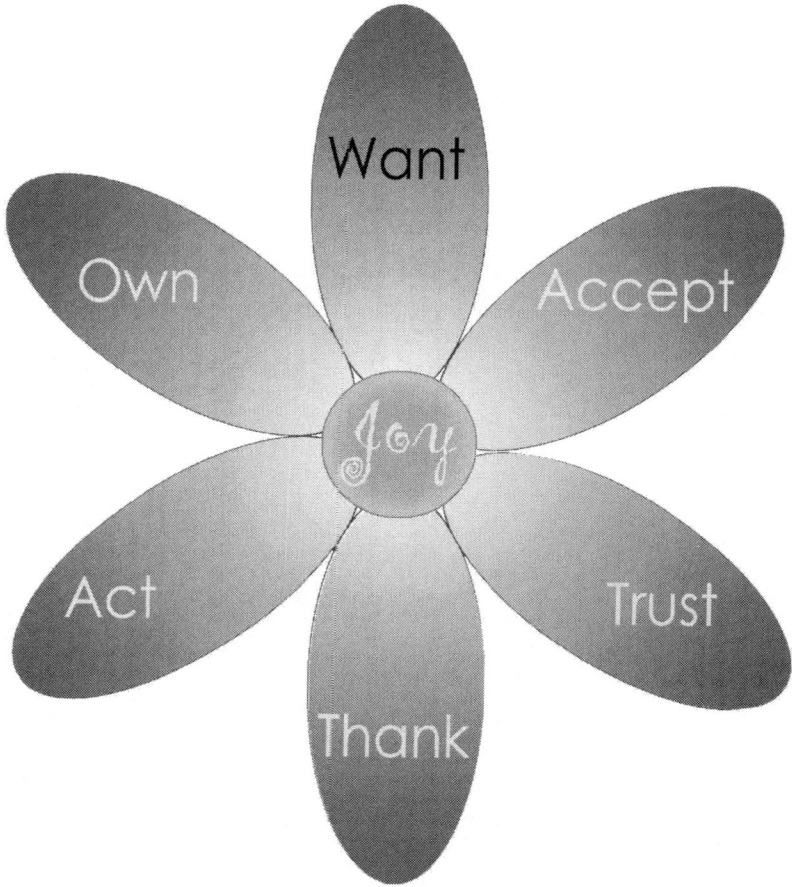

Step 1. Know what you *want*

You decided to face this, well done on your first decision!

Now it's time to define what you know *must* happen in the end. It's what you want so deeply, you just know it's going to happen. If possible, tie this to what gives you joy.

What you are going for is a creating a vision not only of the result, but also of the journey on the way there.

Finding desire in fear

Remember your feelings when you initially received the lab results and the first treatment plan options? These responses are a good indicator of what's important to you. For me I felt that going straight to a LEEP procedure and removing part of my cervix was underserving my individual needs. I didn't know it before that moment, but I realized then that I wanted my cervix whole, and I wanted to explore and talk openly about my needs as a woman and an individual in order to discover treatment options.

> *For the love of God, can we just talk about sex and sexuality.*
>
> *—Girlfriend's response when asked about the importance of opening a public dialogue about HPV and Cervical Dysplasia*

Finding desire through investigation

Maybe you have a strong opinion on an issue but you are wondering if that is based on anything real. If that's the case, you are probably driven to do a bit of your own investigation. *Go ahead and take time to do that.* Use many sources: the internet, your family, friends, someone you know who has gone through this—you can contact me if that feels right.

Be sure to write down your discoveries. After your thoughts are articulated, go back and rate how strongly you feel about each topic. If you haven't written down anything that is a 9 or a 10 in importance to you, keep writing! Keep thinking. Keep investigating. Know what is important to you.

Then, make decisions based on what's important.

> *I could not allow myself (more) medical trauma. Knowing that I had a choice to receive adequate medication while the procedure is being done and the fact that my doctor could refer me to somebody who could do that and it's not a big deal, that's when it started to materialize.*
>
> —*LEEP Patient who had anesthesia for the procedure*

Finding desire in Joy

During my freak-out moment, I realized more than ever that being open and honest with my family, and having their understanding and support is a huge source of joy in my life that I just couldn't do without. Look back to your Joy worksheet and be sure to incorporate that into your vision of healing and wellness.

We need to work on this because it's part of our getting back to together.

—Cryosurgery Patient in five-year relationship
after he healed from genital warts,
and she healed from cervical lesions

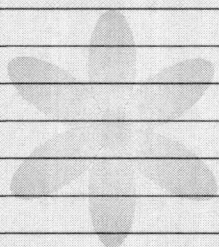
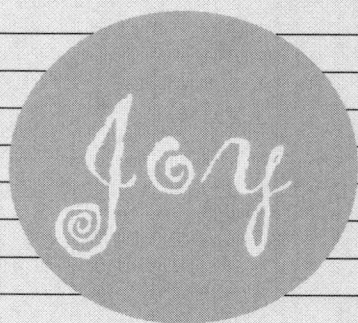

Your Desires

Take a moment now to write down a few notes about what matters to you most. You can come back and reference your notes as a *guide in making informed decisions* on the choices presented to you as possible treatment options.

What you are concerned about? What are your goals?

Revisit your freak-out moment and what you learned from that. Include any constraints you think there might be, like finances or treatment location.

_____

_____

_____

_____

_____

_____

What you just know you *will/will not* have

Is there anything you know absolutely must or must not happen?

_____

_____

_____

_____

_____

_____

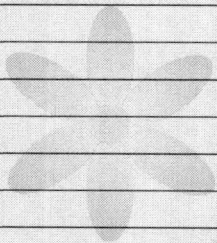

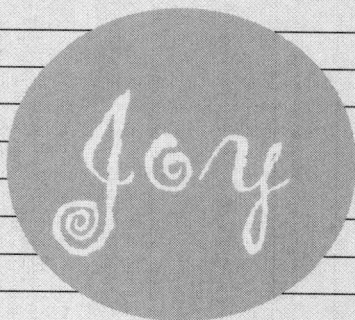

Your gut reaction to the initial treatment plan option

Revisit that moment when your doctor presented the lab results and treatment plan. Is there anything that jumped to mind? Jumped to heart?

_____

_____

_____

_____

_____

_____

How you want to see yourself?

How do you want to feel during the treatment? How will you feel when you are healed?

_____

_____

_____

_____

_____

_____

_____

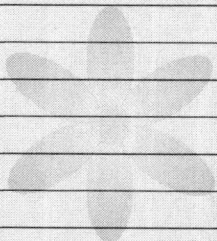

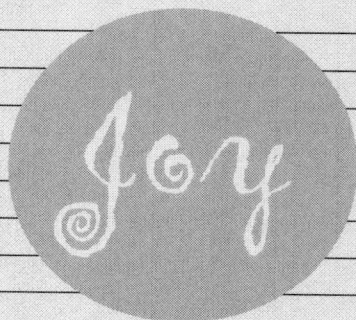

Your additional investigations, discoveries

Your decision

Summary from My Story

- **I *will* do something.** I discovered 'watch and wait' is not a good answer for me. There are alternative treatments and I want to give them a chance.

- **I *will not* be shamed by this** and try to keep it to myself. I want my family to be at peace when they think about my health and well-being.

- **I *will* have my cervix.** I want to savor sexual activities I've found that make me feel truly alive as long as I can, and for now, this involves keeping my cervix.

- **I *will not* have LEEP** unless absolutely necessary. I don't want to pursue a treatment (LEEP) that makes me feel medically underserved as a person.

My decision: My cervix is worth fighting for.

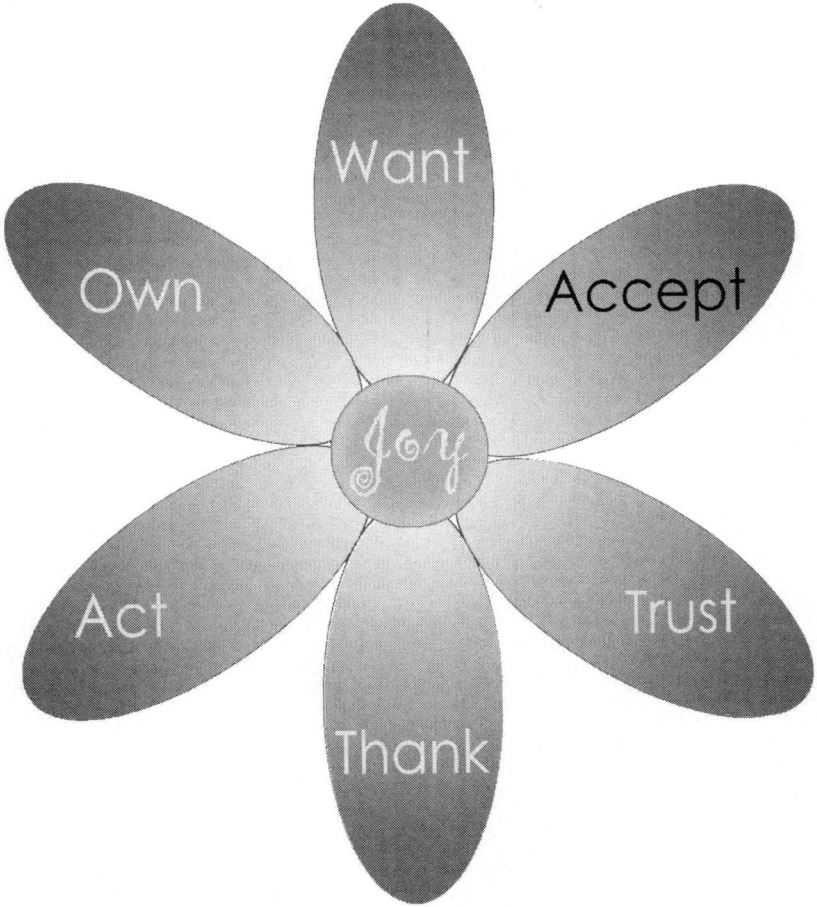

Step 2. Accept where you are now

What is going on in and around you right now? Honest current situation observation is not difficult, since it's things you already know and do right now. The trick? Take time to notice it, as it is—not how you wish it to be, or how you previously thought it was. Acceptance of where you are now will not only motivate you, but it will help you understand your ability to realistically move forward.

Acceptance will ultimately reveal what you believe in. Once you can articulate what you observe about how things really are, then you can consider if you need or want to change anything. Do you believe you may need to let something go? Do you believe you might start something new? Do you believe you can?

Acceptance will also help you realize your superpowers or the power of the situation around you. Is there something about yourself that is just going to shine no matter what? Is there something about the people or the places around you that will affect your path to wellness? Anything that will make the path smoother? These things you want to recognize so you can take advantage of them when you form your healing hypothesis!

Finding acceptance in what you have been ignoring

Because HPV and cervical dysplasia have no symptoms you can feel, it's really easy to ignore. This is strangely reinforced by the 'wait and see' so-called treatment plan and may be a contributing factor to the 'see and treat' approach. Is there anything else you are ignoring that may contribute to your ability to heal?

> *I remember my boyfriend being really embarrassed about it. I think he was pissed that he had warts on his penis.*
>
> —*Cryosurgery patient*

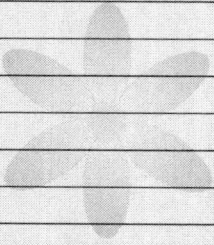

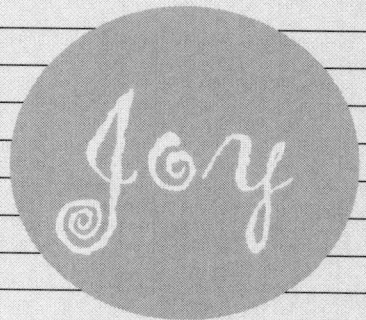

Your Acceptance of the Current Situation

Take a moment now to reflect on what you need to accept either about yourself or about the situation around you. You will want to keep these as reference: *these things will reveal your beliefs and become your superpowers* to incorporate into your healing hypothesis.

How do you take care of yourself?

Observe your own habits in eating, exercising, re-energizing, your work and home environment, your medical care. Note the results and your feelings.

_____

_____

_____

_____

_____

Is there something about yourself that you typically don't share with others?

Observe what you avoid communicating: with people you trust and love, co-workers, strangers. Note why you do that, the results you observe and your feelings.

_____

_____

_____

_____

_____

_____

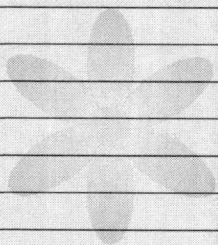

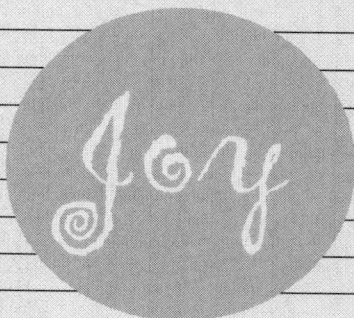

Knowing your diagnosis and potential treatment plan, are you concerned this might be the last chance to do or say something important to you?

Why is it important? Note why you haven't done it so far and how you feel.

_____

_____

_____

_____

_____

_____

_____

_____

Turn your observation and acceptance into action.

Brainstorm actions that honor your observations and acceptance of the current situation.

_____

_____

_____

_____

_____

_____

_____

_____

Examples from My Story

- I *accept* that my immune system is that of an older woman. **I will seek out immune system boosters.**

- I *accept* that my Western doctor's methods are limited and may not serve me well. I suspect the current insurance system may be contributing to that. **I will explore and try safe, affordable alternative treatments.**

- I *accept* that I haven't prioritized taking good care of myself/ my body, even though I still have expectations of continuing physical activities and achievements. **I will put energy and resources into self-care.**

- I *accept* that my alternative lifestyle and associated sex life is important to my feeling alive. **I will ensure my treatment plan has room for an active sex life that is safe for me, my partner and my metamour.**

> *I had to accept the idea that I may be required by the medical industry to change my lifestyle, to change myself.*
> *—LEEP patient when asked if there is anything she had to accept about herself*

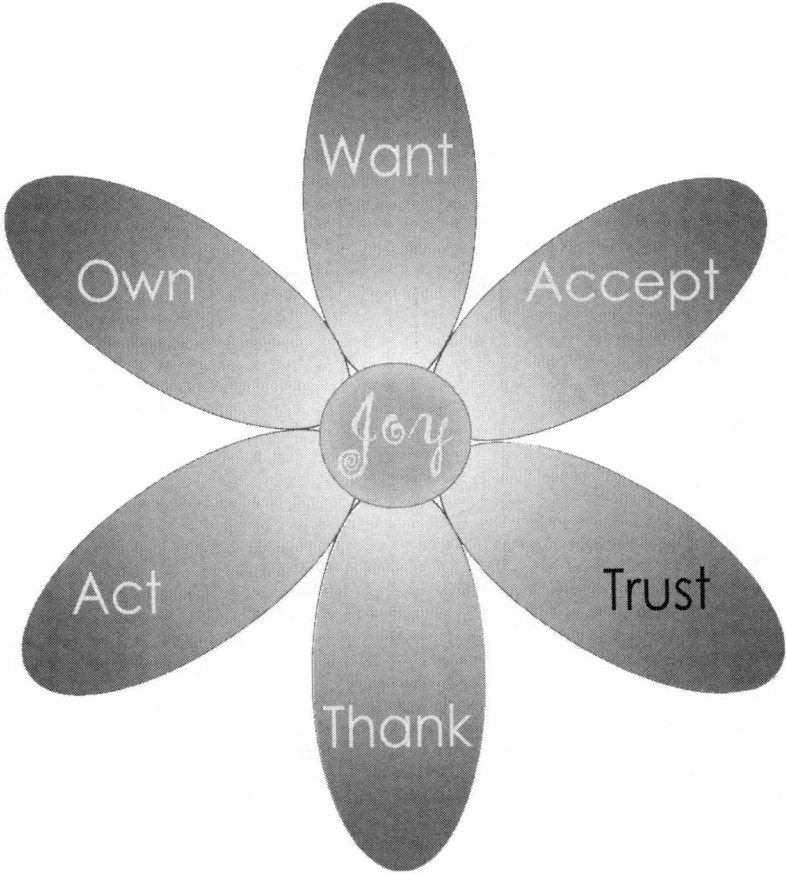

Step 3. Trust your path to wellness

You have done quite a bit of investigation by this point: in both self-reflection and in what's in the world around you. It's time to sum up your findings and make a decision on who you are going to trust and what actions you feel comfortable committing to.

Stating what you trust will reveal the hypothesis of your own healing experiment.

A hypothesis is an educated guess based on what you have learned. Trust is an emotion. Trust is what you are going to offer up to the advisors you have sought out. This is actually a gift you can give yourself. You won't have to concern yourself with *how* to go about healing, your advisors will take care of that. All you have to do is follow what they suggest with full commitment and joy.

> *It is trusting the universe—that the right people are going to come in at the right time. I am grateful that I have that belief. That leads to a sense of security.*
>
> —*Cryosurgery patient*

Your Trust

Take a moment now to reflect on who and what you will trust. You'll want to keep these for reference, because *this is the basis for how you will validate the hypothesis of your own healing experiment.*

Did my advisor ask me what results I wanted?

Observe how your advisor interacts with you and your ideas.

How do you feel about their advice? How will you know when you have realized the desired result?

_____

_____

_____

_____

_____

Did my advisor include my key concerns
in the proposed treatment plan?

Review your Step 1 notes.

_____

_____

_____

_____

_____

_____

_____

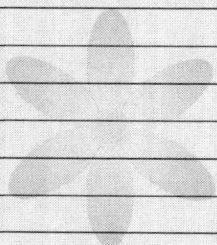

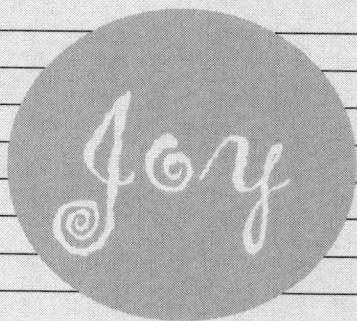

Did my advisor include acceptance of my current situation in the proposed treatment plan?

Review your Step 2 notes.

_____

_____

_____

_____

_____

_____

_____

_____

_____

_____

If there is a problem with the body, let the doctor look over the body. You immediately begin looking at the mind. You see perfect health and you get emotionally involved.

—Bob Proctor, webinar 2017

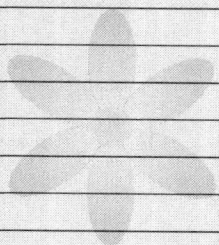

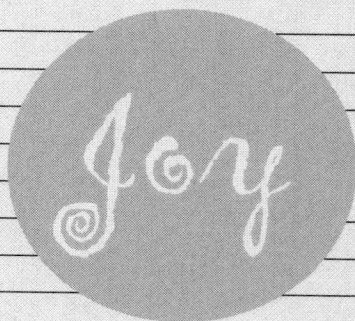

YOUR HEALING HYPOTHESIS

Summarize what you've discovered and decided to form your healing hypothesis.

Given: <Step 1: what you *will* have>

_____

_____

_____

_____

Question: <Step 2: what you *accept*>

_____

_____

_____

_____

Prediction of healing (hypothesis): <Step 3: what you *trust*>

_____

_____

_____

_____

Measure: <know progress and test hypothesis>

_____

_____

_____

_____

Congratulations! You have taken your health and healing into your own capable hands!

If you are noticing your healing experiment is sounding different than my experience, or the experience of someone you know, good on you for taking the time to understand what you really need and want.

Example from My Story

Given: I want to avoid LEEP if I can, I want to proactively do something to progress in healing. I want to keep my cervix whole as long as I can.

Question(s): Why did I not set up that LEEP appointment? Why did learning about yoga practices as healing techniques feel so right? Why are the results from the naturopath's treatment plans so positive? I accept that the standard go-to western treatments do not serve me well at this point, that I believe in breathing as medicine and that the holistic, root-cause treatment approach of the naturopath can be exactly what I need.

Prediction: I believe, given the chance, my body can heal itself. I trust the advice of my yoga teacher and the naturopath, and I believe if I follow their methods carefully, I will heal and think of myself as healthy.

Measure: After I follow the yoga and naturopathic methods for the span of time recommended by the ACCA for cancer screenings, I will go in for Pap and HPV labs and measure my progress.

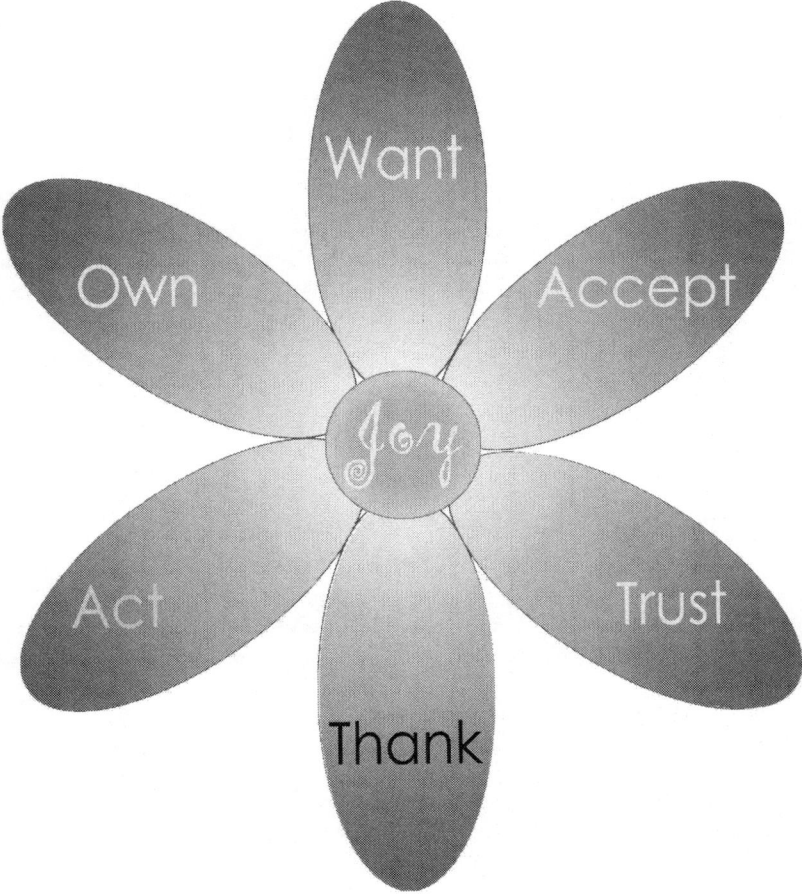

Step 4. Create a vision of gratitude

> If you do *one thing* suggested in this book, this is it!
>
> *Transform all the results you are expect-
> ing into tangible actions of gratitude.*
>
> *Visualize your wellness like it's already happened to you.*

Subtle but powerful! Feeling grateful usually happens at the end, as a reflection of things that already happened. What you want to do is be grateful as soon as possible, be grateful for your healing now and every day.

> *I'm grateful for all those people who took the time to post online. I got to learn and I got to center myself in this whole situation and find out where I belong and be able to predict what I might experience.*
>
> —*LEEP patient*

> *(The nurse) walked me through everything and she said, "I am going to be the person by your side through this."*
>
> —*LEEP patient describes her gratitude for a supportive nurse*

Your Vision of Gratitude

Here's a space for you to jot down notes. You will want to keep these as reference when you do thank-you moment planning.

Brainstorm who you want to thank, and the message you want to deliver.

Think about how this will benefit them.

Who's contributing to your Joy? Removing obstacles? Helping you make decisions? Modifying their schedules? Just listening to you or encouraging you?

_____

_____

_____

_____

_____

_____

What are the details of the thank-you moment?

Picture everything, how you feel, the lighting, temperature and sounds, etc.

_____

_____

_____

_____

_____

_____

_____

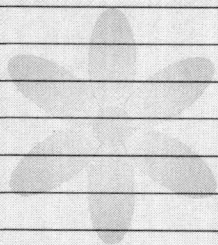

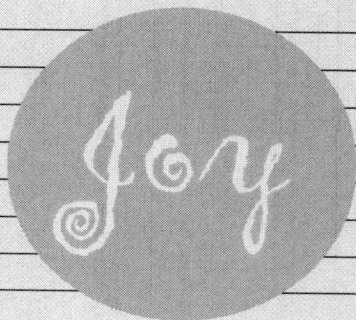

What physical tokens or symbol of personal connection would you like to give?

Revisit the Materials List if you need starter ideas.

_____

_____

_____

_____

_____

_____

_____

_____

What do you need to prepare?

Give context to your thank-you, so they will understand.

How do you describe your goal and their involvement in your realizing your goal? Do I need to make any arrangements for them to be able to receive this?

_____

_____

_____

_____

_____

_____

_____

There is no wrong way to say thank you

When I was a kid, I delivered a thank-you incorrectly. I was with my grandma, and we visited one of her friends. As we were on our way out the door, I forgot to say thank you. So in the car, my grandma scolded me, and told me to march right back up there to the door and say thank you. I was horrified on a couple levels. I was embarrassed I forgot the manners my mom painstakingly taught me. I felt terrible I managed to do something that made my grandma scold me, she never got mad at me! I was asked to bring further attention to all this by doing the walk of shame back to the door of my grandma's friend. How do you do a Sorry and a Thank-you at the same time anyway? Being what it was, I slinked back up to her door, which she was still standing in, and said, "My grandma told me to thank you." This choice to not deliver gratitude with my own intent of appreciation earned me a swat and an ear-pulling back to the car.

I think it was ever since that time, I have always been a bit fearful of expressing gratitude. Clearly, saying thank you the wrong way could get you into big trouble.

As it turned out, it was time for me to let all of that go.

After I delivered that thank-you that day in the meeting room, to people who had no idea why I was thanking them, then to have such an overwhelmingly loving response—I am very sure, if you expect nothing in return, there is no wrong way to say thank you.

> *I feel gratitude that I took a day off afterwards when I didn't need to, because I did need to.*
>
> *—LEEP patient's tip*

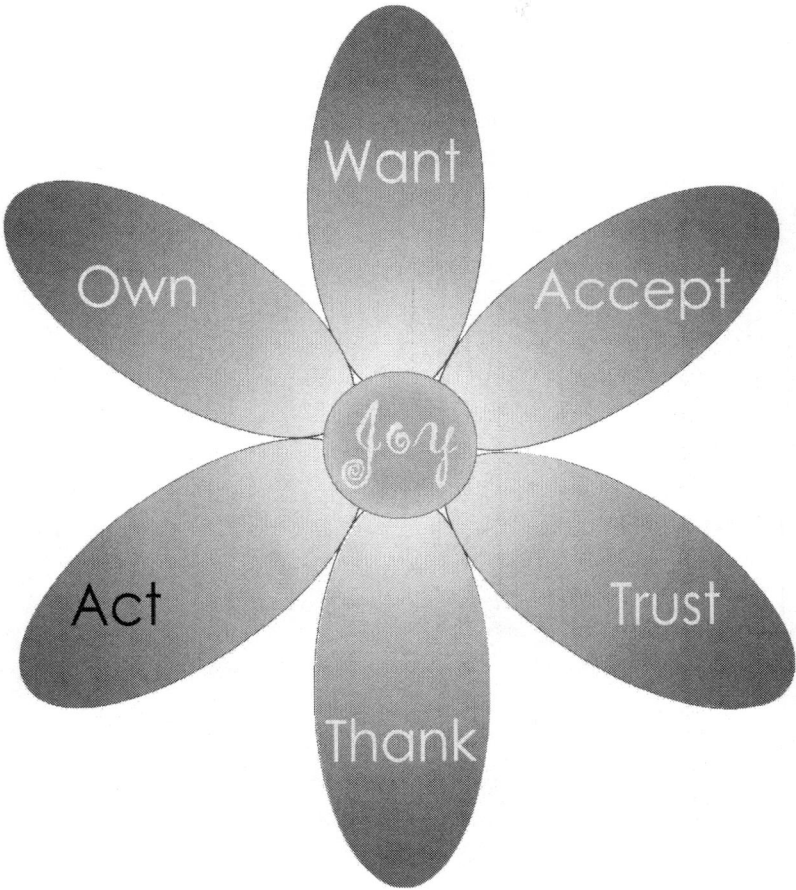

Step 5. Act

It is time to conduct your healing experiment.

This process has been all about making a series of decisions that help you establish commitment: a commitment to step through your own path to wellness, designed by you.

Did you notice along the way, that if you honestly:

- knew what you wanted

- accepted where you are as you are

- trusted yourself and those who are there to help and love you

- felt grateful

- put your joy in the center

Did you notice that with all that, it turns out it doesn't really matter how old you are, the social or family pressure surrounding STIs, HPV or female body parts, or that you freaked out from time to time?

It's incredible what you have accomplished so far.

Now all that's left to do is keep moving forward.

> *It's serious yet it's not serious. You gotta take it seriously. Yet not bring it up.*
>
> *—comment on treatment decision-making from woman with CIN2 lab results*

Your Healing Experiment

Review Your Healing Hypothesis

Note the activities to prove out your prediction.

Procedure 1.

Review Your Trust

List below steps, cycles, materials schedules, etc. Whatever you need to follow the treatment plan you decided to follow.

_____

_____

_____

_____

_____

_____

Materials List

_____

_____

_____

_____

_____

_____

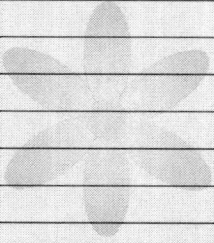

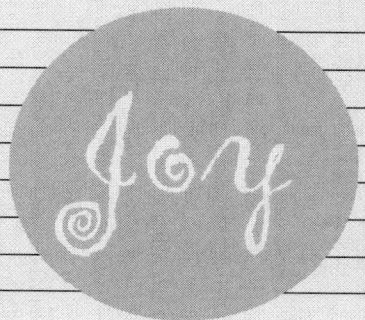

Procedure 2.

_____

_____

_____

_____

_____

Materials List

_____

_____

_____

_____

_____

Gratitude

*Review **Your Vision of Gratitude***
Note how you will fit gratitude activities into your healing procedures.

_____

_____

_____

_____

_____

_____

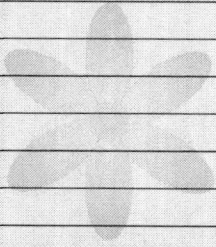

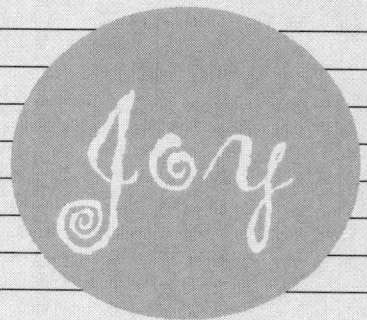

Joy

*Review **Your Joy***

Note the activities, and how they fit into your healing procedures.

_____

_____

_____

_____

_____

_____

_____

Measurement

*Review **Your Healing Hypothesis***

Note how you will fit measurement activities into your healing procedures.

_____

_____

_____

_____

_____

_____

_____

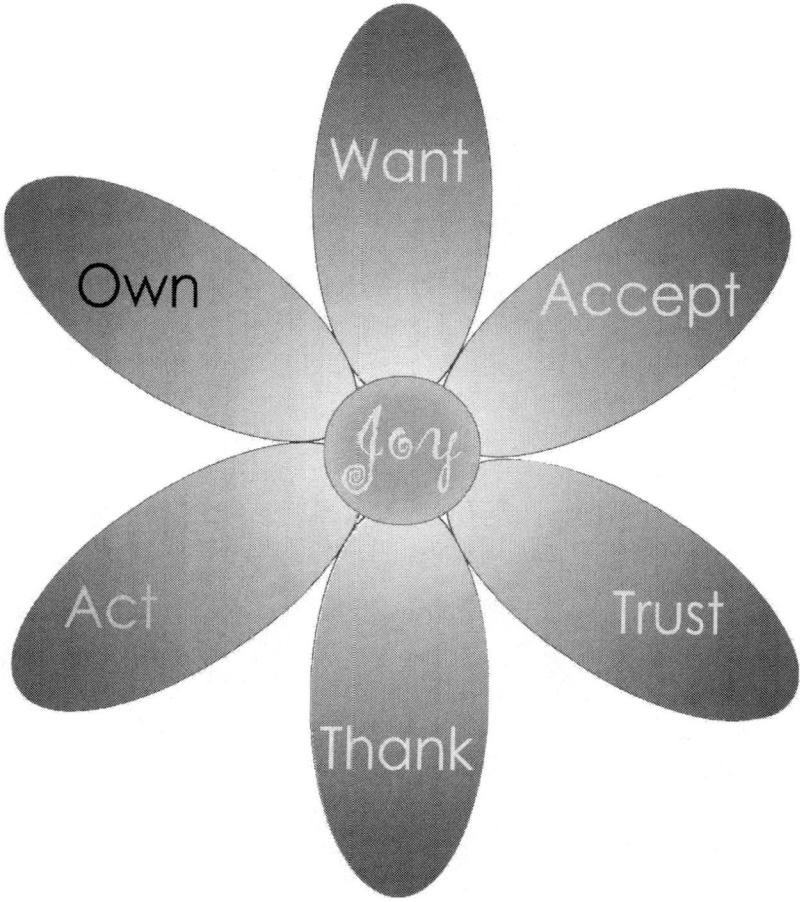

Step 6. Own your new wisdom

Learning I can heal myself was a mind-blowing conclusion of my personal experiment. As I go forward, these are the top three bits of wisdom I carry with me. No matter what choices you make, I encourage you to infuse your own path to wellness with these essentials:

#1 Continue doing what makes you feel alive and whole.

> This is especially important when some so-called experts may suggest you give these things up.

#2 Include tangible acts of gratitude as part of your vision.

> As soon as possible, begin to feel thankful for the results you are seeking..

#3 Grow tolerance into acceptance of where and what you are.

> Observing clearly the current situation will allow you to form a realistic path forward that you can believe in.

Once the healing experiment is over and the hypothesis is validated, this experience is part of us. We are transformed.

What will you do with your discoveries?

I offer my story to help raise awareness of options for HPV treatment and to remind women of their power in choice-making.

—Teresa Marie Novak

Alternative treatment patient with natural cervical dysplasia regression at age fifty— encouraged and loved beyond measure.

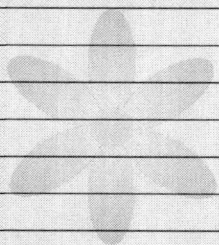

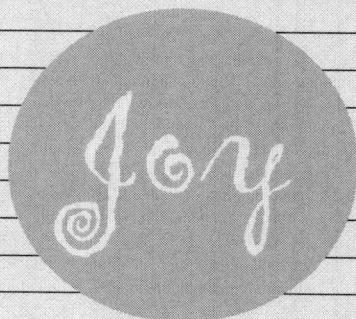

Owning Your Results

Reflect on your experience.

What did you discover? What will you do differently going forward?

How can you pay it forward?

Want

_____

_____

Accept

_____

_____

Trust

_____

_____

Thank

_____

_____

Act

_____

_____

Own

_____

_____

Example from my story

Want: I am healthy.

Accept: I believe through engaged self-observation, I can accept things as they are and use that as the advantage in designing actionable solutions.

I am not alone: 250,000 to 1 million women *a year* are in this same problem-solving position I've been in.

Trust: I can trust my intuition. I can create my own path to healing.

Thank: People around me become my healers.

Act: I can heal myself.

I can designate other people as my healers—without them even knowing it.

Own: I will listen to my body more, and stop ignoring it.

I am contributing to someone's healing and well-being whether I know it or not.

Celebration

> *I've been really good about getting Paps every year. Really good. I'm on my 26th year of getting clear Paps.*
>
> *—Cryosurgery patient*

Materials List

About the Author

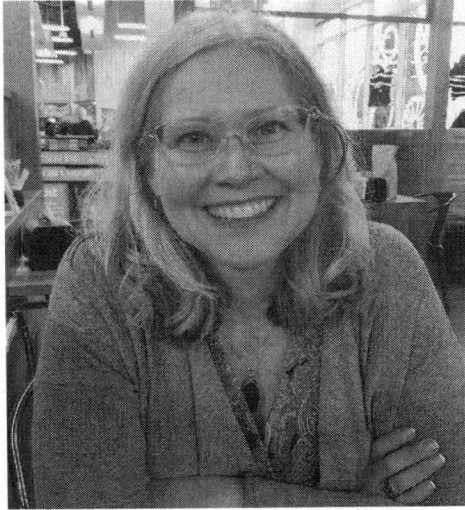

Teresa Marie Novak has been described as 'too kind for the industry' during her day job as an enterprise analyst in software engineering.

Terrie was born in 1967 and the second adopted child of a loving and generous mid-west family. She grew up in Ft. Collins, Colorado and when she wasn't in school or band camp, she was exploring mountain campsites or her grandparents' 100-acre farm in Liberty, Nebraska.

She studied engineering at CU Boulder and finished her undergraduate degree in physics at East Carolina University. In the 1990s Terrie began coding for an educational software company. With this start in tech industry, she made a career of helping people define their problems and desires. Terrie used industry standard methods in systems analysis thousands of times as she led others in creating and implementing processes and products that bring about change.

Terrie learned of the healing power of meditation, yoga and the mind-body connection when she was introduced to the idea by a mental health councilor during treatment for panic attacks and chronic gut and back pain. After she tried naturopathic medicine to heal from HPV and cervical dysplasia and discovered the high statistics associated with over-treatment of LEEP in America, she knew her experience could become an opportunity to educate women about HPV treatment options and the power of choice-making.

This is Terrie's first book, and corresponding courses on the application of the infinity flower transformation process are in development. Terrie self-identifies as solo-poly and has been in a polyamorous triad for over five years, which is a likely topic for an upcoming project.

You can contact Terrie directly at terrie.concept@gmail.com and follow her as Terrie Novak on Facebook and theterrienovak on Instagram.

Thank you, Bear.

References

[1] Approximately half a million LEEP procedures in the United States each year (American Cancer Society).
www.hindawi.com/journals/bmri/2014/875438/

[2] Co-testing
www.nccc-online.org/hpvcervical-cancer/cervical-cancer-screening/

[3] What is HPV
www.hopkinsmedicine.org/kimmel_cancer_center/centers/cervical_dysplasia/HPV/

[4] Stage 0 cervical cancer means the cancer cells are confined to the surface of the cervix.
www.cancercenter.com

[5] Cervical dysplasia can regress.
www.catie.ca/fact-sheets/infections/hpv-cervical-dysplasia-and-cancer

[6] What is cervical dysplasia?
www.hopkinsmedicine.org/kimmel_cancer_center/centers/cervical_dysplasia)

[7] What is LEEP?
www.plannedparenthood.org/learn/cancer/cervical-cancer/whats-leep

[8] Planned Parenthood, a nonprofit organization that does research into and gives advice on contraception, family planning, and reproductive problems.
www.plannedparenthood.org/

[9] I used an alternative name for my hairdresser, at her request, and Sheri is the name of my cousin who was fighting stage IIIB cervical cancer at the same time I was doing my healing experiment. Sheri is a survivor!

[10] See-and-treat overtreatment
www.ncbi.nlm.nih.gov/pmc/articles/PMC4920705/

[11] No data suggest overtreatment is harmful.
www.ncbi.nlm.nih.gov/pmc/articles/PMC3401687/

[12] The importance of the scientific method, according to Bill Nye.
www.youtube.com/watch?v=_tcfyer6dho

[13] For a full description of pawanmuktasana see the Pawanmuktasana Series Part 1 in "Asana-Pranayama-Mudra-Bandha" by Swami-Satyananda-Saraswati. http://www.znakovi-vremena.net/en/Swami-Satyananda-Saraswati---Asana-Pranayama-Mudra-Bandha.pdf

[14] "The most used treatment modality was LEEP, personalized and performed by highly experienced personnel; the 8.8% rate of residual/recurrent high-grade lesions was at the lower end of the 5–30% published rates". www.hindawi.com/journals/bmri/2015/984528/

[15] "Overall sexual satisfaction, orgasmic satisfaction and vaginal elasticity were significantly decreased up to one year following LEEP." www.ncbi.nlm.nih.gov/pmc/articles/PMC4247814/

[16] Eight-angle pose: Astavakrasana yogainternational.com/article/view/eight-angle-pose-how-to-astavakrasana

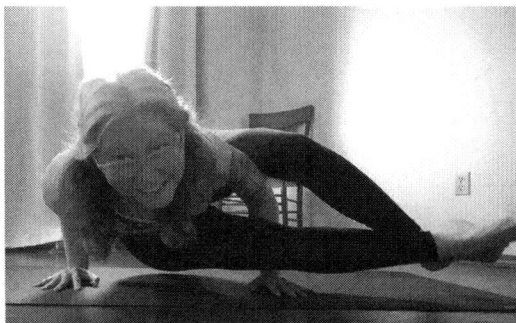

[17] "Naturopathic medicine recognizes an inherent self-healing process in people." www.naturopathic.org/content.asp?contentid=59

[18] Pam died of cancer prior to the publication of this book. She often offered support and encouragement to me as I was writing. I miss her, her smile and her kindness.

[19] "DIM has been shown to help control viral infections, support immune function and reduce certain forms of inflammation." ortwaynephysicalmedicine.com/blog/the-benefits-of-dim

[20] "An increased incidence of cervical dysplasia has been found with low levels of vitamin C (ascorbic acid) in several studies" Romney 1985; Liu 1993; Potischman 1996; Palan 1996; Kwasniewska 1998; Buckley 1992; de Vet 1991; Kwasniewska 1996; Lee 2005.

[21] Green tea extracts in the form of a vaginal delivery and an oral capsule are effective strategies for treating cervical lesions.
drtorihudson.com/prevention/green-tea-and-women%E2%80%99s-health/

[22] What is a vaginal depletion pack?
www.diagnose-me.com/treatment/vaginal-depletion-pack.php

[23] "BDSM is a variety of often erotic practices or roleplaying involving bondage, discipline, dominance and submission, sadomasochism, and other related interpersonal dynamics. Given the wide range of practices, some of which may be engaged in by people who do not consider themselves as practicing BDSM"
en.wikipedia.org/wiki/BDSM

[24] Effects of oxytocin on the female body
www.livescience.com/35219-11-effects-of-oxytocin.html

[25] HPV-16 infective after 7 days
howtogetridofwartshome.com/hpv-and-warts-wiki-guide/

[26] Carrageenan-containing over-the-counter sexual lubricant gels, could block the sexual transmission of HPV.
www.ncbi.nlm.nih.gov/pmc/articles/PMC1500806/

[27] The Gowey Protocol.
www.naturopathsinternational.org/abnormal-papsviral-care.html

[28] Brandie Gowey
www.youtube.com/watch?v=j_bqSRisZPo

[29] Pawanmuktasana Series Part 1
http://www.znakovi-vremena.net/en/Swami-Satyananda-Saraswati---Asana-Pranayama-Mudra-Bandha.pdf